D0117848

GET ME THROUGH TOMORROW

AMERICAN LIVES | *Series editor: Tobias Wolff*

GET ME THROUGH TOMORROW

A Sister's Memoir of Brain Injury
and Revival

MOJIE CRIGLER

University of Nebraska Press
Lincoln and London

Library of Congress Cataloging-in-Publication Data

Crigler, Mojie.
Get me through tomorrow: a sister's memoir
of brain injury and revival / Mojie Crigler.
pages   cm.—(American lives)
ISBN 978-0-8032-5414-5 (pbk.: alk. paper)
ISBN 978-0-8032-6997-2 (epub)
ISBN 978-0-8032-6998-9 (mobi)
ISBN 978-0-8032-6999-6 (pdf)
1. Crigler, Jason—Health. 2. Brain damage—Patients—
United States—Biography. 3. Brain damage—
Patients—United States—Rehabilitation.
4. Brain damage—Patients—Family
relationships—United States. 5. Brothers and
sisters—United States—Biography. I. Title.

RC387.5.C75 2015
617.4'810443—dc23
2014035369

Set in Huronia Latin Pro by Lindsey Auten.
Designed by A. Shahan.

For my mother and father

Driven far off course by the warring winds,
over the vast gulf of the sea—battling home
on a strange tack, a route that's off the map.

HOMER | *The Odyssey*

Just want to be there to help you find your way.
Get me through tomorrow, through today.

JASON CRIGLER | "Through Tomorrow"

PROLOGUE

In the middle of a song, something in Jason broke. Looking out over the crowd that packed Sin-é, the thirty-four-year-old guitarist saw the lights at the far end of the club begin to bulge. He blinked, then squinted, trying to refocus his eyes, but the lights continued to swell until eventually they stretched out over the room, expanding into long glowing blue and white and yellow lines that hovered near the ceiling.

The first two songs had felt normal, as had the sound check, dinner, and the entire day beforehand. Now singer Sandy Bell's voice sounded far away, and the music seemed as if it were playing down a hall instead of surrounding him. Jason checked the pedals, cables, amp, and his yellow Squier Telecaster, a guitar he'd played thousands of times without trouble. The equipment looked fine, as did the other musicians, all of whom Jason had worked with for years. Unable to hear them, he was playing into an abyss, moving his fingers by rote memory of the song. Surely whatever was happening soon would pass.

But the music began to materialize in front of him, each note forming then floating away down a long tunnel. Bewilderment gave way to panic. He threw his guitar over his head. With his hands pressed together like a wedge, he pushed through the crowd to find Monica, his wife. Two months pregnant, Monica had been staying home lately, but tonight she'd wanted to hear Jason play.

His eyes were crossed. He was holding his head with both hands. "I need help," he said.

She led him outside. The night was unseasonably cool for August. Attorney Street rang with New York's late-night summer soundtrack of radios, horns, whistles, and yells, but to Jason it all sounded miles away. Dizzy, unable to keep his balance, he lay down on the sidewalk. Someone placed a folded jacket beneath his head. Monica called 911. While they waited for the ambulance, she knelt beside him.

"What's happening?" he asked, again and again.

She was saying something, but her voice was too far away to hear.

GET ME THROUGH TOMORROW

1

The ringing phone cut through my sleep like a slap.

"Marjorie." I heard my mother's steady, serious voice. "I'm at the hospital with Monica. I think you should get down here. Jason has hydrocephalus."

A dim automatic picture of my brother came to mind: thick and strong. I saw his broad shoulders and sandy brown hair, and I felt his height, six foot one, a part of him known in my neck from looking up at his face. Jason, harmed? The idea lay beyond my reach.

"What's hydrocephalus?" I asked.

"Water on the brain. There's been a bleed in Jason's brain."

Bleed in his brain. A waterfall in his head, dark fluid pouring over a precipice, going where? Questions lined up on the edge of my mind—Why? Will he die? How will he get better?—and hovered there like shadows. My ability to think was diminishing to the speck of one phrase: *bleed in his brain.*

I dialed the number of a car service to take me from Brooklyn to Manhattan. Hollow inside, I was moving like a robot as I dressed. Fear had taken over my body. Now find your wallet and cell phone, said the robot's command center, and I mindlessly complied. Keys. Sweater for Monica, as requested. The ER is cold.

Earlier I had fallen asleep while watching a documentary about the terrorist group the Weather Underground. The film was research for a play I'd written that I wanted to revise for an upcoming production at Carnegie Mellon University. When I'd woken up to let my dog, Lila, out in the garden behind my studio apartment, I'd picked up a message from Monica, who had called while I was asleep. She and Jason were at St. Vincent's Hospital. It looked like Jason had a bad ear infection.

"I don't think it's anything to worry about," she'd said.

I had listened to her message in a groggy haze. For weeks I'd been working long hours in the script department at NBA Entertainment, preparing for the Athens Olympics, which the NBA was producing the basketball competition. In addition to writing announcements and introductions, the script department created documents that synchronized the production and broadcast teams. My colleagues included two documentary filmmakers and another playwright. In between TV production jobs—award shows, holiday specials, political conventions—we worked on our own projects. A few of my plays had been workshopped at theaters in New York and San Francisco. The Ensemble Studio Theatre, with the Alfred P. Sloan Foundation, had awarded me commissions to develop the play that was going to be produced at Carnegie Mellon.

Later I would think that if I'd picked up the phone when Monica called, everything would have been different. Later still, I would realize that it made no difference. The truth was, I wanted to believe Jason had an ear infection. I could not believe he was in trouble. Innocent or in denial, I had gone back to sleep.

Outside, the car was waiting. At 4:00 a.m. Prospect Avenue was deserted: rows of low brick tenement houses and, on the other side of the street, a commercial linen supply service, now locked up and quiet. I directed the driver to St. Vincent's but after a block asked him to turn around. I had forgotten the sweater for Monica.

Back in the car, I hugged the sweater, a heavy black hoodie with white letters, BROO, on one side of the zipper and KLYN on the other, a Christmas present from Jason and Monica in 2001.

It was August 5, 2004.

As the car sped through the empty streets, I prayed. *Bleed in his brain.* I knew nothing about the brain or how it could be hurt, and my ignorance felt as terrifying as going to the emergency room in the middle of the night. I looked out the window, wondering if this moment was going to be the line in my life marking before and after. As we crossed the Gowanus Canal, I thought, Wait and see.

Impatient, I told the driver to let me out on Thirteenth and Seventh Avenue. I thought the ER was between Twelfth and Thirteenth, but it was a block farther south. I ran. The streets were dead. No cars. No people. I seemed to be the only thing moving.

When I entered the ER, Monica and Muma (my mother's family nickname) walked toward me, crying, and draped their arms around me.

"Is he dead?" I asked.

"No," they said. Not dead. But close.

A nurse asked if I wanted to see Jason. Most likely—though I wouldn't realize until later—he was offering me a last chance to see my brother alive. I was led to a bay in triage. Wearing jeans and a red zippered sweatshirt, Jason looked like he was sleeping. His chest rose and fell with heavy deep breaths. He seemed so much his normal self that I didn't feel moved to speak any more than I would have upon seeing him take an afternoon nap. I had asked Muma and Monica point blank if he was dead, but I didn't think he was going to die.

On my way out I stared at his white tube sock, wanting to draw my finger up the center of his foot. EMT training, which I'd completed a year earlier, had taught me that this was a test—but for what? The EMT textbook's section on head injuries floated before me, its pages maddeningly blank. I left without touching his foot, but back in the waiting room I told Monica, Muma, and Rop (our name for my father) that I had done it and that Jason had responded correctly. I don't know why I told this outright lie, except that I wanted desperately to have proof of what I could only hope was true.

The attending neurosurgeon—I'll call him Dr. Glass for his large wire-rim glasses—approached us, flanked by two residents. As we rose to greet them, I thought, It is proper to stand when receiving terrible news. Introductions were made, all in relation to Jason. Wife. Mother. Father. Sister.

"His neurological prognosis is not good," said Dr. Glass.

"What does that mean?" we asked. "How can you tell?" We were like a Greek chorus, speaking as one, or one of us speaking all of our thoughts.

Dr. Glass said that Jason's response to a neurological test was poor.

"What was the test?" we asked.

The doctor had pinched Jason's chest, and Jason had moved his arm—showing that he felt the pain—but he had stretched his arm away from the pain instead of reaching toward it, as someone with healthy neurological functioning would do. I could picture this gesture. I had seen it in people with limited mental ability. A basic answer to stimulus. Not sophisticated. But Jason was sophisticated. He was intelligent. He had *so much* in his brain.

We asked the hard question. "What are his chances?"

"He might not survive," Dr. Glass said, adding, "I am cautiously optimistic."

I could feel all the parts of Jason that hung in the balance: his wry sense of humor, his compassion, his street smarts, his pride and determination, his love for Monica, his thrill at becoming a father. I remembered sharing a taxi with him soon after Monica's first of two miscarriages, which had happened while Jason was in Los Angeles on tour with Erin McKeown. The night we shared the taxi was his first gig and his first night back in the city, and though I had spoken to him and Monica over the phone, it was the first I had seen him since the miscarriage. I had watched him, however, on a KCRW webcam when Erin and her band played a set on Nic Harcourt's show, *Morning Becomes Eclectic*. The camera swung back and forth, giving me a grainy image of Jason, and I ached to think how sad he must feel, yet he had shown up. The other people in the cab got out at their apartments, and then Jason and I were alone. "I'm so sorry about the baby," I said, and his voice choked with sorrow as he replied, "Thanks, Moe."

When Dr. Glass and his residents left, I collapsed, bawling, moaning, as sobs jerked out of me. Rop was crying too. Muma was murmuring, "No, no, no, no." Softly, into her phone, Monica said, "Daddy?"

I pictured Jason moving his arm in response to the pinch, only capable of that single simple answer. *I feel*. Was that all there was left of him? Loss pulled on every piece of me. Would this be the extent of his communication? Would he live but on the far side of an impenetrable wall, beyond our attempts to decipher his sounds and movements?

I feel may be the most information a creature can convey or it may be the catalyst for a symphony.

One other family had been with us in the ER through the night. Their three faces reflected a gratitude that they had their problem and not ours. I had been aware of their gaze as first we sat in terrified anticipation and then we crumbled in shock and grief. I knew the other family was watching the seismic change taking place in our lives, and their witnessing this moment made me hyper-aware of us, of what kind of people we were. The woman in the other family caught my eye and said, "We pray for you."

Yes, pray, said a voice in my head. Because your tears are doing nothing to help Jason.

I went to the small bathroom off the waiting room, locked the door of a stall, and knelt on the grimy yellow-tiled floor. I put my hands together and bowed my head.

"God?" I said aloud.

As if in response, the toilet behind me flushed. Its automatic flusher had been triggered by my movement. Still, the timing was perfect. A tiny laugh arose inside me, like a single firecracker bursting in a vast and desperate darkness.

2

He was always there. In the bunk above me. Ahead of me on the shiny slides of Central Park playgrounds. Walking at night down West Seventy-Fifth Street, the soles of our pajamas scraping the sidewalk, our parents towering above as Keeper, our husky, pulled us toward rowdy Broadway, where music and grown-ups spilled out of taverns and Moondog, the homeless Viking, shouted from church steps and where once we saw a thief rip a string of pearls from the neck of a blonde in a black fur coat. Jason was there beside me running down the grassy hill, Superman towels for parachutes. Charging me fifty cents to go down the slide in the bedroom we shared, whose picture window looked out on our untended garden with its ivy-covered walls, white butterfly chairs, and, in the winter, Snow Mountain. When it rained, Jason would sit under an umbrella in the garden's open doorway, whereas I would cocoon, curled up on Muma's homemade Marimekko window seat cushions. More often than not, we shared a bedroom, with bookshelves dividing the space. In his half, x-Wing and TIE Fighters hung from the ceiling by fishing wire; my half was the Moe Office, publisher of the *Moe Office Press*, each issue made by folding newsprint into my boxy gray Royal and typing around empty boxes in which later I'd draw pictures or glue photographs. Though I couldn't see him I could always hear him: the squeak of the swivel chair, the rustle of a page turning, the slide of fingers re-creasing the comic book's fold.

In a photograph taken when we were five and three, Jason is in a red cape, red briefs over blue tights, red and yellow *S* emblem sewn onto the front of his blue shirt, chin thrust out, shoulders squared, gaze to the distance. My costume is less elaborate, a purple cape over my gingham jumper, enough to play the game. Jason is Superman. I am his knock-kneed, dewy-eyed audience; his first fan.

When I was born, Jason couldn't pronounce *Marjorie*. The closest he could get was *Mojie*, and that odd, funky name stuck because it suited me, a girl with a gap between her two front teeth and long braids running down either side of her head. Many people have known me as Marjorie, an elegant if old-fashioned name given to me in memory of my great-grandmother. But inside I have always felt more like a Mojie, and in the divine, truth-telling way that two-year-olds have, Jason was the first person to recognize that.

When he was twelve, Jason started playing the drums. At sixteen he discovered the guitar. He practiced for hours. I understood Jason's discipline and determination because I knew him as his sister, and siblings hold nothing back. In each other's presence they rage, wail, pout, obsess, triumph. They learn each other passively, over time: rhythm of gait, depth of sighs, body's sounds and smells and even taste. Siblings witness. They come to know what makes the other seethe, what makes the other laugh. This is how I knew Jason. Absorbed in his interests—first acting, then drawing, then everything else falling away for music—Jason affably put up with the rest of life but wasted no time returning to what he loved most. Growing up, I saw how he cared—the loyalty, the sweet concern, the ferocious underlying drive—which is to say, I saw how he lived: true to his heart, hardworking, led by love.

In the ER the intensity of my response surprised me. I had never before felt this surge and pull of grief, which, with the same helplessness, disorientation, and lack of air, felt like being caught off guard by a big ocean wave. But there was more to it than that. As adults, Jason and I hadn't been all that close. We kept each other informed, saw each other occasionally, rested assured that the other was there, somewhere. We did not turn to each other for advice or problem solving or outpourings of the heart. Both of us had friends, colleagues, lovers who knew us on a more daily basis. Even as I sobbed I was perplexed. I loved him, yes. I feared for him, yes. And something more. At the time I could not begin to understand. I could only be carried. There was no choice but to give myself over to the feelings roiling inside me. And this in itself was telling. My deepest connection to Jason lay beyond thought or reason. It belonged to a part of me that even I couldn't claim to know.

3

Dr. Glass wanted to drill a hole in Jason's skull. The bleed had caused a blockage between two ventricles, the sacs in the brain that produce the cerebral spinal fluid (CSF) that lubricates the brain and spinal column. Because of the blockage, the ventricles weren't draining properly. They were filling with CSF and squashing Jason's brain inside his skull's fixed confines. Dr. Glass wanted to create a ventriculostomy—an opening in the ventricle—whereby a thin tube would drain excess fluid from the third ventricle into a container outside Jason's head.

"Will drilling hurt his brain?" we asked. "Will it damage his ability to play music?" Dr. Glass promised that he would avoid the part of the brain that stores musical knowledge.

When the operation was repeated a week later, I would ask the resident to avoid the same area, and he would give me a small smile and say, "We're careful with all of the brain." He would tell me there was no way to protect specific skills or knowledge, making me realize that in the ER Dr. Glass had only told us what we'd wanted to hear.

Since Jason would go from the operating room to the Neuro-ICU, we moved from the ER to the hospital's main waiting room. The sun had come up. People were starting to arrive for work, coming through the revolving door with coffee and newspapers, swiping their security cards, hustling to catch the elevator before its doors closed. Night had conformed to our emergency, the quiet streets and near-empty ER feeding my perception that our situation was the sole thing happening in the world. Now normal life was resuming but without us. It appeared strange, separate, as if taking place on the other side of a window.

I called Caroline Laskow at the NBA. I'd known Caro since our undergraduate days at Stanford University, and Jason had composed the score for her first documentary. Through tears I explained why I wasn't coming in. My voice wobbled, but as I laid out what we knew and didn't know, I began to feel steadier. Caro said she'd relay the message to the producers, already in Athens, whom I had been planning to join in two days.

"Do you think you'll be able to go?" she asked.

The odds at that moment felt fifty-fifty. Maybe, just like that, Jason would be fine.

Outside, the bright sunshine, the cloudless blue sky, Seventh Avenue's morning bustle, the very date and time, belonged to a new world where every single thing was marked with *Jason*. His absence.

St. Vincent's was only a few blocks away from the five-storey walk-up where Muma and Rop had lived when they moved from California to New York in 1965, earning free rent as their building's superintendents. They were newlyweds then and recent graduates of the University of the Pacific, where Muma had studied music therapy and Rop played piano in the conservatory. ("When I hear your father play," she once told me, "I remember why I fell in love with him.") After earning their master's degrees—she from Columbia Teacher's College, he from the Juilliard School—Muma started teaching while Rop began accompanying opera singers, including luminaries such as Leontyne Price.

By the time Jason and I were born, in 1970 and 1972, Rop was the musical director of the Goodspeed Opera House, a theater in East Haddam, Connecticut. In addition to overseeing orchestrations and arrangements and helping to choose, cast, and rehearse the shows, Rop conducted the orchestra in which Muma played the cello. Because Muma was also teaching in New York and because they preferred the New York schools for Jason and me—and most of all because they liked living in New York—we shuttled between city and country: summer in Connecticut, winter in New York, and spring and fall we rode back and forth every week. That was our happy crazy schedule until they divorced, in 1988, marking the start of an era so different from preceding and subsequent years it might have belonged to another lifetime. Where once they laughed, now they seethed. Their easygoing confidence gave way to brittle fear. My soft daydreams were displaced by a hard seasick confusion. They left Goodspeed, and soon after, Jason and I left for college.

It took us a decade to snap back, to remember. After the divorce Muma started hosting Thanksgivings with open invitations for friends and colleagues without dinner plans. Thirty or forty people would fill her apartment, a boisterous mash-up of her friends, Jason's friends, and, after I returned from California in 1999, my friends too. By then Muma and Rop were reconnecting, tentatively, realizing they could reach beyond the divorce to other pieces of their past, for they had, in many ways, grown up together. One November, after several years on the road conducting national touring companies, Rop was home on Thanksgiving. Muma invited him to dinner, where they were cajoled into playing a duet. I stayed in the kitchen, not wanting people to see my tears. At Jason and Monica's wedding in 2001, I found myself with him and our parents, laughing in a way—wholly, gut wrenching, time stopping—that made me feel like we had resurrected the better part of who we used to be.

In recent years Muma had found love again with Fred Siegal, an immunologist specializing in AIDS research, now working at St. Vincent's HIV Center. Fred was why, when the ambulance paramedics asked Monica if she had a hospital preference, she'd said, "St. Vincent's." Now, after a quick tasteless breakfast, Muma, Rop, and I were following Fred through a maze of hallways to his office, which he offered as a refuge from the main waiting room, where a dozen of Jason's friends had gathered in something too much like a hangout, a happening, the loud group oblivious to the waiting room's other occupants who were quietly dealing with their own crises. "What have you been up to lately?" one friend casually asked, but chitchat was a forgotten foreign language. I said something in response, but all I heard was the hollowness of my voice. How could I put the past five hours into words? How could I explain that everything else was irrelevant?

Dr. Glass called Fred's office to say the surgery had gone well. The ventriculostomy was in place. He'd reviewed scans of Jason's brain, and though the images were too blurry with blood to determine anything, he had some thoughts. I took notes:

AVM—high risk of rebleed. arterio venous malformation
tumor
cavernous angioma

tectum

1. operate?
2.

a. shunt
b. angiogram

aqueduct of silvius
3/4 ventricles

We were looking at three potential culprits. AVM and cavernous angioma were different kinds of irregular blood vessels. Cavernous angioma seemed like the best option to hope for. Behind the tumor loomed cancer, and the AVM held the highest risk of bleeding again.

The hemorrhage had occurred near Jason's tectum, which, I would learn later, is the roof of the midbrain, a primitive piece of anatomy that belongs to the brain stem, the controller of life-or-no-life actions such as breathing and heart beating. *Tectum* made me think of tectonic plates shifting and colliding to cause an earthquake, and it didn't seem far off to think that an earthquake had taken place in Jason's brain.

An angiogram—an X-ray image of blood vessels illuminated by a high-contrast dye—would tell us what had caused the bleed. But because some people have allergic reactions to the dye, angiograms require a patient to be stable, which Jason was not. We would have to wait and hope that whatever the cause, it would not strike again. Perhaps the angiogram would tell us to operate. But since the bleed had occurred deep inside Jason's brain, traditional surgery (i.e., cutting through tissue) might do more harm than good. The second option was not to operate. What then? The second option was a blank.

The bleed had caused a blockage between Jason's third and fourth ventricles, a narrow passageway known as the aqueduct of Sylvius. The path of water through the forest, I thought, five long-ago years of Latin attempting a translation. In fact, Franciscus Sylvius was the seventeenth-century anatomist for whom the passageway was named. The term had nothing to do with *silva*, Latin for "forest."

For now the ventriculostomy would keep Jason's ventricles right sized. But this was not a permanent solution. The external drain could infect easily. After a week it would need to be moved. If the aqueduct of Sylvius didn't clear up on its own, a shunt would be installed. We didn't like the idea of a shunt. We wanted the problem gone. We wanted Jason back.

4

Broken, grotesque, Jason slept, still sedated. A fat white tube ran through his mouth and down his throat. A respirator was pumping oxygen into his lungs. His head, half-shaved where the drilling had taken place, was flecked with spots of dried blood and stamped with a row of dark stitches. A thin tube ran out of his skull to a clear cylinder half-filled with cerebral spinal fluid made murky red by the hemorrhage. To prevent him from pulling out the respirator, his wrists had been tied to the bed rails.

I had seen Jason injured before. Very young, we sat in a bathtub, surrounded by floating toys. For his make-believe shaving, Muma had given him old bladeless razors—except this was not one, which he ran up his arm. She and Rop rushed in, and Jason was carried away.

There was the time he returned from a bike ride, entering our summer cottage holding his arm while telling me he'd fallen on the steep driveway.

"I'm going to lie down," he said, and I turned back, unperturbed, to my game of solitaire spread across the kitchen table.

"He's still sleeping," I said when Muma called between the matinee and evening shows, and someone from the theater came and took him to the doctor, where his broken wrist was set and cast.

For a dozen summers we rented that cottage or one of the other nine at Bennett's Poolside Cottages, a modest old country resort nestled among forest, family farms, and century-old cemeteries. There were three acres, a swimming pool with a slide, a playhouse, a swing set, a rope swing, and a dog named Good Boy. Three children in the Bennett family plus Jason and me and the handful of kids with a mom or dad working at Goodspeed made up the gang that spent its days in the pool and on the swings and ventured to the strip mall up the road for pizza and candy and (my weakness) the stationery aisle at the pharmacy. We played chase late into the night, though the dark corners in which I hid frightened me, as did the loud lonely sound of my breathing as I waited for the roving mob to find me, and sometimes I went home early while Jason ran with the older kids. At Bennett's a Rockette taught me how to swim underwater. At Bennett's a short tough boy brought me, at dinnertime, to watch his snake eat a mouse. At Bennett's Jason chased or was chased by a friend around the swimming pool, Jason wearing long flippers, which was at first funny, clownish, part of the challenge, and then plain stupid when the tip of a flipper caught, bent, sent Jason face first onto the pavement. Seeing the white bandages covering his face, I wondered—no doubt influenced by late-night reruns of *The Twilight Zone* and *Alfred Hitchcock Presents*—if he would heal so radically changed as to be unrecognizable. But he emerged the same as before. Same mole on his right cheek, same blue eyes, same slightly loose lower eyelids, same face that contorted into ridiculous grimaces and then like rubber returned to a resting expression of patient readiness.

Years later in New York, again just the two of us, teenagers after school, Jason greeted me at the front door, holding his hands above his head. "Do we have any Band-Aids?" He had been trying to adapt a thick strip of embroidered cloth into a guitar strap when the scissors slipped.

"In the little bathroom," I said, brushing past him.

"You might not want to go in there," he said.

Blood was splattered across the sink's white bowl, the doorknob, the tiled floor, the blue-and-white wallpaper, the medicine cabinet, the toilet seat, the mirror that hung over the toilet to make the closet-sized room seem bigger. I found the Band-Aids. Still, he and Muma went to the ER that night because we could see in the cut his bone.

His injuries were crises. My only serious medical claim was a ventricular septal defect, a hole in my heart, which sounded more like an explanation than a medical condition. It meant penicillin with every visit to the dentist and a biannual two-hour bus ride to Columbia Presbyterian for an EKG until I was twelve, when the doctor said, "You're one of the lucky few. It closed up on its own."

Bleed in his brain was different from anything we'd known. Instead of bloody flesh, broken arm, busted face, sliced finger, here was an absence of information. No cast, no Band-Aids, only waiting. Until when?

The group of friends had migrated upstairs. They were traipsing in and out of the one-room, six-bed Neuro-ICU. I wanted to punch the man who joked, "Jason, you look so sexy." Another stood staring with his mouth hanging open. Why did they need to see Jason now? But who was I to ask them to go away? Jason was an adult, after all. How much sway did his family have over who came near him? I could imagine him saying, "Sure, Moe, let them stay." But their presence, perhaps simply their number, brought disorder to a situation that begged for tranquillity.

"You need to leave," Muma said at last.

Home briefly to walk Lila, I called one of the NBA producers. "I totally understand," she said when I told her I couldn't go to Greece. They had already bought a plane ticket for my replacement.

Heading out the door to return to St. Vincent's, I grabbed a pocket-sized red-trimmed black notebook, a miniature version of a present Jason once gave me for my birthday. The satisfying paper and binding and weight had prompted me to ask where he'd bought it: Ming Fay Book Store on Mott Street, where I had since bought all my notebooks. I'd picked up this one in anticipation of my trip.

Part of me didn't want to take the book. But if I didn't start now, writing would become impossible. I would want to remember minutiae. There was too much to hold in my head. Already some details—quotations, descriptions, medications—were gone. If I didn't take notes, I would regret it. But writing was difficult. I felt distracted on a profound level, as if a cloud had settled over my thoughts.

August 5, 2004. Half of me denies this is happening. I look up and around and think, This is happening to Jason, to Jason, my hero. Don't let your mind run wild because fear shoots fast and far. The world looks entirely different when one's brother is in the ICU.

The next morning, tattooed and pierced Nurse Bea reported that during the night Jason slid down the bed until his elbows were past the restraints, then pulled the respirator out of his throat. Also, she said, his eyes were open.

We cheered. Here was the Jason we knew—stubborn, determined, triumphant Jason, whose response to the theft of his new eight-hundred-dollar amp had been to open the Yellow Pages and call every used instrument shop in all five boroughs.

"If you see the amp," he'd asked each place, "please call me."

"I've got your amp," said the man who called. "I'd be happy to sell it back to you."

Furious, Jason called the police, who set up a sting. Jason went to the store, and when the owner offered a price for the stolen amp, Monica—already there, pretending to browse—signaled the undercover cops to make an arrest. Thus Jason reclaimed his Princeton Reverb.

That was the Jason we knew.

But when I saw him, my heart lurched. He had been intubated again because Dr. Glass wasn't sure he could breathe on his own, and his eyes, though open, were rolling in different directions. His irises were clearer and bluer, the whites whiter, as if his eyes had been washed clean. They expressed total innocence, as if he were too consumed with figuring out the situation to bother with fear. What if his eyes were stuck like this? Vaguely I knew that vision involved the occipital lobes at the back of the brain, but what that actually meant and how Jason's eyes could be fixed seemed a black hole of cause and effect. We had Jason—but how much?

Waking, he gagged on the respirator.

"It has to be there for now," I said. "Can you try to relax?"

He settled back into the pillow. I dug the red-trimmed black book out of my bag, stuck a pen in his hand, and held the little notebook where he could feel it.

"Tell me," he wrote.

The letters were Jason's. The *m* was the same I'd seen on every *Happy Birthday Moe* and the *e* hung ajar in his familiar script, which had always seemed to me boyish, laid-back, a little messy. I thought of the connections in his brain forming the words, the muscles in his hand coordinating to write, the cut-to-the-chase curiosity of his command: Tell me, because I know something's wrong.

We told him what we could. A bleed in your brain. We don't know what caused it. We don't know, we don't know, we don't know.

5

Friday afternoons Jason and I would meet Muma at the Stephen Gaynor School, where, in addition to teaching, she created the music and computer programs. Sometimes we waited downstairs; other times we yanked shut the stiff brass folding gate of the ancient elevator and rode to her fifth-floor classroom.

Like a gun, Stephen Gaynor's dismissal bell signaled the start of our race. We hustled a few blocks to the downtown subway, Muma carrying her cello in its heavy hard case. "You know you're on the C," she told us, "if at Fifty-Ninth Street the wall is on your right. If it's not, switch to the train across the platform."

Once, Jason and I were without her and forgot to look for the wall until it was too late. "We're on the wrong train," Jason said.

I suggested backtracking.

"No." He sounded weary at the idea. "It's okay." On crowded, busy Sixth Avenue he seemed to sniff out the right direction, then said, almost under his breath, "We go this way."

From the Penn Station subway stop Muma, Jason, and I would trot along the underground passageway, past the garbage can storage cage, past the video arcade with its upside-down sign, up the infernally steep brass staircase, past the lockers and loiterers, into the main room forever under construction. We didn't wait for the big black board, fluttering with arrival and departure information, to flip our train's track number. Instead, we charged downstairs to the cramped smoky Arrivals Lounge, filled with people who didn't look like they were waiting for trains, where we checked the board for the train from Washington (which was the train to Boston) or found the conductors on break, who recognized the woman with two children and a cello and told us the track.

In the train's restroom—or dressing room, which some cars featured then—I changed from school uniform into jeans, stuffing the wool tunic into my red nylon duffel bag. Every now and then a passenger complimented Muma on her well-behaved children. More often, she silenced us with a demand—*I want you both on best behavior*—delivered in a tone that turned my stomach cold.

Rop picked us up in Old Saybrook, and we drove straight to Goodspeed for the eight o'clock show, buzzed through the stage door with the password *orchestra*, stepping into the dark cement stairwell, as cool as a cave, heading either downstairs to the green room—and from the green room down a tight spiral staircase to Rop's office—or upstairs to the dressing rooms, or up another flight to the house, orchestra pit, and stage left. On Fridays we raced to reach the theater on time. Sometimes the train was late and the stage manager had already called places. Then Rop and Muma sprinted to the pit. Countless times the four of us won this steeplechase, whose victory was sounded by the first notes of the overture.

Jason and I fought and teased each other mercilessly, but we were also allies, loyal by necessity, the only other one who spoke the language, understood the protocols, knew the routes between our worlds.

Goodspeed—always overly air-conditioned, always smelling like the mints, lemon drops, and pastel candies sold at the gift shop—premiered one new show each season, but its mission was reviving old musicals. Their titles signaled a bygone era: *Tip-Toes*; *The Five O'Clock Girl*; *Oh, Kay!* They were stories of high society, mistaken identities, statues that came to life, safes that opened only with the right soft-shoe routine. The score, written for a twenty-piece orchestra, would be arranged for about nine stellar musicians, many of whom doubled or tripled on instruments. The house was small, with warm clear acoustics. No one wore a microphone. The performers were mesmerizing, not only the leads but also the character actors and the chorus, which always had one or two tap dance numbers that stopped the show. To hear the music and see the dancing—to be so close to it, to experience that live—was mind-blowing. Jason and I saw some shows thirty or forty times. We watched them from every angle, from the balcony steps to the orchestra pit. Or we listened through speakers in the green room, where, between the Saturday matinee and evening shows, long tables and folding chairs were set up and the members of the cast, crew, orchestra, box office—many of whom came back year after year—together ate dinner prepared by the guild. Once everyone was seated with food, someone would start a round of applause for those who had made the meal.

Or the show was no more than a muffled soundtrack as we used the electric typewriter in Rop's office to create our own scripts, usually backstage capers or orphan stowaways on transatlantic steamers. We taped the pages to the back of a couch behind which we crouched, holding aloft our Muppet puppets. Santa had given Kermit and Animal to Jason, Rowlf and Miss Piggy to me, and these assignments were right: Jason was leader and wild thing; I was laid-back and diva. When Muma and Rop emerged after the curtain call upstairs, they became our audience downstairs.

Following the Sunday matinee, the four of us piled in the car and drove to New York, Jason and me in the back seat, surrounded by knapsacks and duffel bags, eating McDonald's, watching the highway as the sky turned dark. Monday morning we suited up for school, Jason in a jacket and tie, me in my navy blue uniform.

After our parents' divorce we became full-time New Yorkers, though really before that identity could take hold we graduated high school and went off to college, and then some of the worlds to which we had traveled disappeared from our lives, leaving memories like a dream to which only he and I could testify.

6

August 6. A doctor asked Jason his name.

"Jason," he rasped.

"Do you know where you are?"

"Hospital."

"Do you know what year it is?"

"2004."

"Do you know what city you're in?"

He looked at the doctor with a worried expression.

August 8. He asks how we are. He wants to hear gossip. He wants to know which of his friends came by. He wants pizza. (He got broth and orange-flavored ice.) His eyes are still crossed. He has ringing in his ears, which Dr. Glass says may never go away. He remembers 2004, August, all of us, the events of Wednesday night, but not St. Vincent's, the nurses' names, or what procedures took place, even after we tell him.

We could do nothing but wait. Wait for the blood in his brain to wash away. Wait for a scan to show what had caused the bleed. Wait for him to wake up. Wait upon his words for clues—was he more alert today than yesterday? More talkative? More himself?

On the heels of Jason's admittance, a social worker met with Monica to apply for Medicaid and SSDI (Social Security Disability

Insurance). Even though Monica's job as a graphic design artist at an educational publisher gave her and Jason health insurance, St. Vincent's knew the insurance company would deny some of the claims. Medicaid, they hoped, would pick up the rest of the bill. In pushing these applications, St. Vincent's was doing something we could not—namely, taking a long view of the situation.

We thought this would be a short episode. Jason would bounce back and we would report the experience as a kind of What I Did on My Summer Vacation. "It was scary," I imagined myself saying, "but everything worked out." I couldn't contemplate what would happen if things went awry. The alternative to Everything Worked Out was an abyss so foreign that I didn't have the words or pictures to imagine it, and so I tried to believe that it didn't exist.

"He'll be ready to play in a few weeks," Monica was telling people with whom Jason had work lined up.

Because I had planned to travel in Greece after the Olympics, I had a month free before I was due back at my other job, as an attorney's secretary, which gave me health insurance and let me take leaves of absence for writing gigs. Muma was on summer vacation from the Columbia Preparatory School, where she'd taught for the past decade. Rop, who had recently been on the road conducting productions of *Ragtime* and *Some Like It Hot*, was home with no plans to go out of town. Monica took off first one day, then another, then another. After two weeks she had to return to work. She came to the hospital in the evening and raced over when procedures required her signature.

A friend suggested that for financial help Monica contact Musi-Cares, a philanthropic arm of the Recording Academy, the organization that gives out the Grammy Awards. The application required a complete list of every band with which Jason had played and every album on which he'd recorded. But Jason was hired by word of mouth or people hearing him. Résumés didn't mean much in his world. With dozens of musicians sending Monica details of their work with Jason, she pieced together a history of his career.

The final document, which garnered some funds, was long and impressive—no surprise. Jason had been a working musician for many years. After college he'd moved back to New York and worked at the Foundation Center while playing guitar at night, asking himself if he should be an expert amateur musician or try to make a living at it. "There are so many bad guitarists out there," he said when he quit the day job. "I just have to be good. If, on top of that, I'm a nice guy who shows up on time, I think I'll be okay."

He was right, which is not to say that it was easy. But his hard work paid off, and in time he established a reputation as a talented, dependable, generous sideman, playing with John Cale, Marshall Crenshaw, Linda Thompson, and many other singers and songwriters who were famous, not famous, or not yet famous. He'd toured throughout the United States and Europe and appeared on *Late Night with David Letterman*. He was a fixture in the clubs on the Lower East Side.

Often when Monica left for work in the morning, Jason would be sitting down to practice, and when she returned he would be in the same place, still going. Once, to challenge himself, he retuned his guitar to an obscure tuning used in British folk music, requiring him to transpose every song he played. He approached a piece asking not only what he could add but also what could be stripped away. What was necessary? How to get inside the song?

Starting in the 1990s, as computer software advanced, Jason belonged to a group of industrious, do-it-yourself musicians who were creating polished original independent albums in their home studios. They recorded in each other's apartments during the day and performed together at night.

Sometimes he would book a gig and recommend other bands that he played with for earlier and later slots, meaning he was onstage from 7:00 p.m. until 2:00 a.m. At one point, feeling stuck, he consciously chose to say yes to any gig, regardless of his opinion of the band's sound. Soon he had more offers than he could accept, and, far from sacrificing his taste, he was playing with performers he'd admired for years. Some Fridays, with bassist Rob Jost and drummer Robert Di Pietro, he provided dinner music at the Blue Fin in Times Square. They would bring charts and sight-read a repertoire-expanding panoply of songs, from jazz standards to Brazilian sambas to the Beatles.

I ran into him in Times Square on a Friday afternoon, one of those moments when New York is simultaneously colossus and hamlet. He and the Robs were killing time before the Blue Fin, and I went with them to Manny's, where they tried out instruments and someone bought guitar strings and I laughed at their pre-show banter, whose playfulness and reciprocity would resurface in their music. Robert Di Pietro told me about the time he'd taken a gig far below his ability, "a step back," as he'd described it to Jason, who had replied, "Forward or back—it's a step."

But there was also the time an engineer accidentally recorded over Jason's guitar track, the worst time for such a mistake, the track having been an extraordinary solo, and hearing the engineer explain what had happened, Jason punched his hand through a window. He had this side to him too, a heat in his blood that sometimes boiled over.

In the downtown music scene Jason met Monica, who was designing posters and album covers and starting to write and sing songs of her own. The night they met, they rode the F train back to Brooklyn. Afraid she would never see him again, Monica asked if he gave guitar lessons. He did. Soon they had formed a band, calling it Goats in Trees because Monica had seen a picture of tree-climbing goats and thought, A goat in a tree is as crazy as me in a band. Soon they were living together. Soon they were married.

One patient in the Neuro-ICU was a man who had been found by the police, mugged and beaten, no identification. The nurses christened him Butter and called him George. They were waiting to see if anyone came looking for him. No one did. He lay in his bed, intubated and unconscious. He was dying alone, without even his name.

We met the other patients and their relatives, who shared our roller-coaster energy as well as the fervent desire that this episode end quickly and take its place in family lore. How about that time Jason was in the hospital! It would be a scary story with a cheerful conclusion because didn't life turn out that way? Wouldn't everything be all right?

The Neuro-ICU was so small that if one patient needed privacy, all visitors were asked to leave. In the windowless waiting room we read the *Times* or *New Yorker*, finished the daily crossword puzzle, watched whatever TV program was on. Often it was the Olympics, where I had planned to be, and I wasn't upset to have bowed out, but, especially during the basketball competition, I felt dislocated, a vertiginous sense of *I thought I'd be there but I'm here*, as if I were in a car that had taken a turn too fast and my inner compass was still reconciling the change in direction.

We got to know the nurses, in part because we were a family that filed its stories by character. In a desperate twisted way we thought that if the nurses liked us, perhaps they would take extra special care of Jason. Mostly we needed them to translate a quick brusque comment by Dr. Glass, to tell us how Jason fared at night, to give us his latest numbers, such as temperature, intracranial pressure, and white blood cell count. (Increase in ICP meant probable swelling in his brain; WBC spike indicated infection.) The nurses told us about their days off, their complaints about the hospital, the significance of their tattoos, and we read the nurses' demeanors as if they were portents of a smooth or difficult future. And, as if someone had spiked our coffee, we laughed, overtaken by hilarity in the same way that alone I would cry and later see red dots of burst blood vessels in the skin around my eyes.

We already had our own silly intrafamily vocabulary and not only nicknames but nicknames for nicknames—I could be Marjorie, Mojie, Moe, Moegger, or Moegger the Doegger. Some stories and jokes hung around for years, their punch lines regularly trotted out for renewal. Jason had a habit of buying himself a Christmas present, wrapping it, placing it under the tree, then feigning surprise when he opened it. "What's this?" he would say, waiting until the rest of us were numb with coffee and waffles. He read the card straight. "To Jason, from Santa." Opening the present, he'd exclaim—the very picture of Christmas joy—"No way! I always wanted this album! Thank you, Santa!"

We never let go of a good malapropism, as when—another Christmas—Muma picked up a heavy gift, saying, "This weighs a fortune." Our humor must have been influenced by the vaudeville routines that peppered Goodspeed's shows, which Jason and I had memorized and recited—

"Do you feel like a cup of tea, sir?"
"No, I don't feel like a cup of tea. Do I look like a cup of tea?"

Laughter was part of the reason Monica had so quickly felt like family. There was the birthday or Mother's Day when the five of us met for brunch in Brooklyn and I mentioned that I was practicing piano études by William—somebody. I couldn't remember the last name of the composer. "Shatner," said Jason, who was, like Monica, a devoted *Star Trek* fan. "The William Shatner Études," he said, laughing so hard he could barely walk. When Jason laughed, he abandoned himself to it, laughing not just because something was funny but because funny struck him completely, and when he lost himself like this, there was no way not to join him.

As children we'd teased each other relentlessly. For a few years, in our twenties, we stopped, perhaps thinking we'd outgrown it or perhaps the divorce killed everyone's sense of humor or perhaps it didn't work when he was in New York and I in California. Sometime after I'd moved back, one of us threw a barb, the other returned, and we volleyed, falling into our old routine, except unlike when we were young and thought that teasing had agency, that it could settle something, that it *mattered*, now we were lighter and more absurd. We revisited classics like "Muma, who's your favorite?" and radically reinterpreted the standards, as in our operatic version of "You're the problem." For us the tease was not just a jab but a test of endurance. The answer to "Who's your favorite?" and "Who's the problem?" lay in who lasted longest, who could endure the pointless ridiculous endless exchange without going berserk. Our teasing, which used to provoke tears, screaming, pushing, and punching, now led to laughter, with Rop, Monica, and Muma joining in.

In the hospital, when Dr. Glass asked, "Who is the president of the United States?"—a standard question to determine a patient's general orientation—Jason sighed heavily before answering. "Unfortunately," he said, pausing as if he hated to admit it, "it's George W. Bush." When asked for the thousandth time to lift a finger—to gauge his basic muscle command—Jason raised his middle finger. "The Great Meltdown," he called the bleed. We were delighted. Surely humor was a sign of higher brain functioning. If he could crack a joke, we figured, what couldn't he do?

During the long hours of waiting, we wondered which stars would play us in the Hollywood blockbuster version of our story. We held heated debates on whether Viggo Mortensen or Matt Damon was a better fit for Jason, whether Jane Fonda or Susan Sarandon for Muma. The laughter rose when Rop, asked who would play him, said, "Robert Redford," as if we were fools not to see this obvious choice.

"What about Natalie Merchant for Monica?" someone said.

"Natalie Merchant isn't an actress," argued someone else.

A shrug. "It could be her debut."

"Clint Eastwood for Rop?"

"Too old."

"We'll cast him in his younger years."

"Madeline Kahn for Muma?"

"Madeline Kahn is dead."

Laughter all around. *Dead!* As if that mattered.

7

August 9. The drain for cerebral spinal fluid was raised higher, and Jason became sleepy and illogical. His body is not reabsorbing the CSF. He thought he was in the Southeast, and when asked "Are you in a library, a hospital, or a supermarket?" he chose supermarket.

August 10. Muma, Rop, and Fred are talking to doctors at other hospitals about more aggressive treatment. I hadn't even thought about that—what to do, where to go from here. Just hadn't occurred to me. My mind isn't working. Jason whistled a little tune. I have total dread in my heart.

August 12. They moved G. Butter to the ventilator floor, where he will be breathed for until he dies. In the flood two days ago, two people in Queens died getting out of their Nissan. A downed power line electrocuted them. And there is Jason, eating his orange sherbet, reminding us it's 2004, August.

George Butter's terrible lonely end stunned me: mugged, beaten, *breathed for,* done. I wasn't unfamiliar with tragedy. One of Goodspeed's stage managers had stepped off the train in New Haven, had a heart attack, and died on the platform. A number of actors we'd known had died of AIDS. After the ashes of one were scattered in the Connecticut River, a tall wrecked woman turned and looked right at me as she moaned, "That's my brother." In 1994 cancer took Mark Sicher, Jason's close friend since first grade. When Mark died, at twenty-four, he and Jason were sharing an apartment in the East Village.

Now my brother had nearly died, still might die. That ending was quite possible. Or—what? How else might the story play?

To my surprise, my dreams, usually cryptic shards of strange narratives, were direct and lucid. Here was Jason, playing guitar with Monica. Here was Jason, mad at me. Here, on August 14, was me understanding that without us, Jason would not recover:

I dreamed I was in a dark room with a table full of older white men. I'm going to Athens after all, I announced. You are? one of them said incredulously. What about your brother? He's stabilized, I said, but my gaze was cast downward, and I knew I was abandoning Jason to a permanent state of confusion.

At first talking about Jason seemed helpful, healthy; then it proved exhausting, as I felt compelled to answer all questions and didn't want to sound depleted or too emotionally wrought to talk. By acting as if this were a manageable situation, one that could be discussed, I thought it would be so and offered, in lieu of the oft-requested prognosis, a multitude of facts to serve as some kind of scaffolding for hope. But each little piece of information—CSF, ICP, WBC—required definition and contextual explanation. It did not occur to me to limit these conversations. "What do the doctors say?" people asked over and over, searching for certainty, but this question wanted an impossible answer. His condition was too blurry for a prognosis. Jason's future lay not in the doctors' crystal ball but in each passing second he remained alive.

Bleed in his brain. There was no one to blame. No drunk driver. No regrettable mistake. It just happened. And so, although fear had become my constant companion, anger was absent.

But when a website went up reporting on Jason's medical progress, I erupted. The site included a place for people to leave comments. If people wanted to write publicly about Jason, that was their business. But broadcasting his daily status seemed like an incredible violation of privacy. Then a friend, from her vacation in the Caribbean, called Muma. The friend, who was on Jason's email list for upcoming shows, had been sent a link to the site—the first she'd heard Jason was in the hospital. "What do the doctors say?" she pressed Muma, who didn't want to explain, from the beginning, what was going on, but did.

The site, which was taken down, was borne of good intention by people who wanted to help, who felt helpless. But it missed a particular, uncomfortable reality. Even as I hoped this would be a short-lived injury, when I looked at Jason's crossed eyes or heard him say he was in a supermarket, I knew—in an abstract way—that he might take a long time to heal. The image Dr. Glass had given us, of Jason moving his arm away from the pinch, still haunted me. What if his life was that limited? Or what if he could no longer play music? Another story I'd collected concerned a mathematician hit in the head who could no longer calculate but became a successful speechwriter. While such a change would be shocking, the story gave me comfort. The man had adapted and survived.

No one could predict when Jason might come home. No one could say how he'd be tomorrow. We could only show up and try not to think too far ahead and find ways to get from one moment to the next. And wait.

8

He fell.

He had been sitting in a chair in the Neuro-ICU, per doctor's orders. A person can lie in bed only so long before the skin begins to break down, meaning it falls away in patches, and because circulation slows, blood clots can form, move to the heart, lungs, or brain, and block one of the finer vessels there.

Transferring Jason from bed to chair was a delicate procedure requiring two nurses. The first supported Jason, who walked as if he were crossing the deck of a tempest-tossed ship. The second protected the ventriculostomy, catheter, and IV line while also wheeling a vertical metal pole to which were attached bags of fluid and the container of CSF, now no longer cloudy red but clearer than air, the lubricant of the mind totally transparent, invisible but for the faint delineation of its surface. The two nurses proceeded slowly, in tandem, no sudden moves, no surprises.

The first time Jason sat in the chair gave us a rush of relief and exhilaration. Despite his tubes and hospital johnny and sack of urine hooked on the side of the chair, to see him sitting was to gaze upon a wish almost come true. His body wasn't hidden under a sheet, and he sat with his usual posture, a tall man slouching slightly, both relaxing against the chair's right angles and, by his very height and substance, dominating the furniture. Perhaps we were immoderately eager, seizing upon this image of Jason as a sign that everything was going to be all right—he would heal and go home and in six months become a father. Or perhaps our fantastic belief gave us a confidence essential to our situation, a kind of faith that depends not on reality but merely on its own existence.

We heard the crash from the waiting room, a loud prolonged catastrophic sound of metal falling on a cold floor and the free fall of a six-foot-one man. We ran to the Neuro-ICU, but the nurses hustled us out and closed the door.

Left unattended, Jason had tried to stand. He'd wanted to go to the bathroom, forgetting or unaware that he was wearing a catheter. With his damaged sense of balance, he'd fallen over. On his way down his head hit a wall. Miraculously, the ventriculostomy stayed in place, but later I saw a red bump, and I wanted to scream and cry with rage that he of all people should have a bump on his head.

But I didn't scream or cry. I kept that inside, afraid my distress would make matters worse. Besides, against whom would I have railed? It was inconceivable to me to be upset with the medical staff. But Bea was surreptitiously reading *The Lovely Bones* while on shift. Sitting at the nurses' desk, she'd slide the book out from under a pile of papers and read while pretending to be doing something else. When she was needed, she'd slide the book into its hiding place. I was afraid to call her out or tell on her. What if she retaliated by neglecting Jason? I couldn't believe she was doing something wrong. In my desire to like her, and for her to like us and take extra-special care of Jason, I had convinced myself that she was a good nurse. She had to be a good nurse.

While we waited on Jason's improvement, waited to learn the source of the bleed, I became preoccupied with normally forgettable objects, such as the automatic revolving door at the hospital's entrance, which halted unpredictably, an utter failure of efficiency, maddening at best and torturous when I was in a hurry. I puzzled over the design of the waiting rooms, with their intentional blandness, the innocuous framed reproductions and stiff loveseats that transformed into anyone's living room.

I wanted the receptionist to know me because a friendly greeting from her meant the gods favored Jason. The security guard with an acne-scarred face looked familiar. Had I seen him elsewhere, or was I imposing closeness? Or did I simply have nowhere else to focus my thoughts?

Lunch acquired monumental importance. If I perfectly satisfied my hunger, the day would tilt in the right direction, which meant that Jason would be all right. Buying lunch every day felt extravagant, but the indulgence seemed justified. I could look no further than Jason to know that life could end in an instant—so, eat well.

August 18. I dreamed Jason asked me, "Moe, what the hell happened?" and I started to explain but was interrupted. Two nights in a row I wake up thinking I'm going to vomit.

When I wasn't at the hospital, I was at home. Behind my studio apartment was a garden, which had been a junkyard when I first moved in. My landlord ("Ma-*jor*-ie," he called me, in his Greek accent) had turned one of my two windows into a door—actually two, storm and screen, the latter a lovely slice of country in New York—which opened onto a wooden deck and the yard below. I'd spent one whole summer cleaning out the garbage that had for years been thrown over the chain-link fence from the small parking lot next door. Candy wrappers, soda cans, beer cans, motor oil bottles, keys, underwear, and an infinite amount of broken glass. A cat's skull, shotgun shells, someone's stash of empty vodka bottles. Typewriter keys, marbles, at least fifty cat food tins, several cat travel cases, and television packaging foam that had been duct-taped into a pathetic but functional cat house. Mohammed, a neighbor, told me about the old lady who used to live in my apartment. She'd had over twenty cats coming in and out of the three-hundred-square-foot studio. When the woman's Social Security check sat untouched on the mail table in the hall, Mohammed knocked on her door several times, then went through the basement to the backyard and climbed on a chair to look in her window. She lay dead on the floor. The cats were eating her toes.

A ct scan confirmed that despite the fall, the ventriculostomy was still in place, so Dr. Glass proceeded with a plan to clamp the tube in order to test whether the blockage in Jason's aqueduct of Sylvius had cleared. If it hadn't, the ventricles would balloon, press against his brain, and he would become drowsy and unresponsive. Then an internal shunt would be necessary. Now at Day 13 since the hemorrhage, already the ventriculostomy had been switched from one location to another. There was a limit on how many times it could be moved. I pictured Jason's head with hundreds of holes, an absurd and horrifying image, the same nightmare I'd harbored when doctors had amputated my ninety-year-old grandfather's infected foot and I had wondered if they would continue to chop off parts until he was no more than head and torso.

On the day of the planned clamp, part of the ventriculostomy tube's external daisy chain disconnected. The tube hung from Jason's head, an open pipe, exposing his vulnerable brain to all the filthy contaminated bits that float in common air.

No one knew how it happened. The nurses estimated two minutes lay between their discovery of the break and the last time a nurse could remember seeing the tube in place. But who knew? Bea, after all, was absorbed in a book.

Maybe Jason was shifting in bed and disconnected the tube himself, the nurses said. As if he should have known better.

When Dr. Glass told us about the tube—hours after the fact, in the late afternoon—my mind started spinning like a gerbil's wheel. I was desperate to turn the clock back, to undo the previous eight hours. When I looked at the waiting room chairs, I saw not steel and fake leather but bacteria and germs, and the air appeared cloudy with floating granules of poison. Early on someone had told us,

"When you're sick, the worst place to be is a hospital." The meaning of the remark had eluded me. Wasn't a hospital where you got better? Now I understood: if you're vulnerable, if you're exposed, if your ventriculostomy disconnects, you lie at the mercy of any number of potential infectors.

Despite the mishap, Dr. Glass had gone ahead with the plan. In a few short hours Jason had descended through drowsiness into a deep sleep, completely unresponsive to our attempts to rouse him. All day we had hovered in a state of wait-and-see. Were the ventricles readjusting, or were they failing the test? At lunch I'd watched him become increasingly incapable of cutting his food and lifting his fork. "Do you want me to help you?" I had asked, and he'd nodded. Feeding him as if he were a child was awkward and strange, but he didn't have the strength to do it himself. Muma had broken down in tears, begging him, "Jason, it's your mother, say *something*," and I'd felt furious at all sides of the situation: his condition, her desperation, and now, Dr. Glass.

Why had the doctor gone ahead and clamped the tube? Shouldn't we first have made sure the disconnection hadn't caused any problems? I didn't understand, but I kept my mouth shut. Haughty Dr. Glass intimidated me. If I stayed quiet and still, Jason would get well.

A friend, hearing about the fiasco, rolled his eyes as if to say, "Hospitals suck," and I snapped, "Don't do that," wanting to protect my image of these doctors and nurses as Jason's saviors. I thought if I rooted for them hard enough, Dr. Glass and his team would be heroes.

Talking about Jason became even more difficult. People would ask how he was, and I would answer, and they would say, "Can I put you on hold for a minute?" One friend said, "What happened, if you don't mind my asking?" and then, hearing the answer, began to moan loudly. I wondered if people thought talking was "helpful" for me, cathartic, if they saw these calls as a therapeutic gesture on their part, the idea of which made my skin crawl. Nothing was helpful except Jason's good health. Some friends explicitly "checked up" on me, asking if I'd been outside. Yes, with the dog. But for *myself?* "Promise me you'll do something outside that will make you sweat," one friend demanded. I didn't like this notion of personal care that seemed ripped from the pages of a women's magazine. If, when I wasn't at the hospital, I wanted not to jog or sweat or be outside but to stare at the wall, that felt like a perfectly acceptable option. I had no illusion that I could feel all right.

August 19. I waited hours for two minutes with Jay. Oh, Jay.

August 20. There is the patient with no discernible issue who pads through the hallway in pajamas and bathrobe looking as if he has misplaced the remote. We see him emerge from the elevator. We see him shuffle along. Yesterday I might have seen him with a valise, leaving. There is the yeller who hollers at the top of his lungs. "Disoriented," a nurse explained. His words are unintelligible. His throat will be sore. He yells as if a life depends on it, as if calling across a canyon. Perhaps he is calling for someone to save him. Does he think that person can hear him?

August 21. Jason improves—shakily. And—seizures. Little ones. Petit mal. Still. Will there be an end—an end in which we are all alive and happy? God, I pray so.

Petit mal: translated by my rusty French as "little bad." Little bad seizures, in which the patient looks fine but loses consciousness, differ from grand mal seizures, in which the patient convulses.

Jason could be seizing, then wake up, say hello, and seem quite himself. He seemed to be improving and declining simultaneously.

One afternoon, after hours of watching him sleep, I left, planning to go home, but detoured into the Strand Bookstore, lost in the stacks until Rop called. Jason had woken up. I ran to St. Vincent's, ran because, unlike in the ER, now I knew this could be my last chance to see him alive. And if I said yes to his cause every time, my devotion would be rewarded—when, how, by whom was not for me to know.

"He's just drifting off," Rop said when I arrived.

"Jay!" I said, my heart still pounding from the sprint. "I ran all the way here, and you're falling asleep?"

"Hi, Moegger," he said softly as his eyes closed, and I left a second time, crying on the F train, spent and grateful for those two words.

Anticipating the trip to Greece, I hadn't been out of the city in months, so I borrowed Muma's car for a weekend and drove south with Lila. We hiked some of the Appalachian Trail, swam in a cold river, and crossed the long battlefields at Antietam, where nettles stung my legs. At night we slept in a treehouse at the Maple Tree Campground. On my way home, in a near-empty diner, a waitress read everyone's horoscope from *Reader's Digest*. Mine: "Try to see the good in a difficult predicament."

When I returned I went straight to the hospital for the last visitors' hour. Monica and Muma smiled when they saw me, saying, "It's been a great day." Jason had stayed awake for several hours and said a couple of words. But I was jarred at the sight of him, weak and damaged. The trip had given me an outsider's point of view. By the next morning my perspective had readjusted, and what had startled me the night before was not as significant as the words he spoke, however few, and the movements he made, however small.

9

After Muma and Rop divorced, Muma dated a man I despised. Nevertheless, I recognized the courtship as a golden opportunity and one fall day came home with a notice off the school bulletin board. A teacher was selling puppies, one of which the boyfriend bought for us in a doomed attempt to win me over. Being an English teacher, the seller had given the litter names from Shakespeare. Our little golden retriever was MacDuff before he became simply Willie. The dog stayed; the boyfriend soon was gone.

Through Willie, Muma and I befriended a regular morning group of dogs and their owners who met in the Central Park meadow off Ninety-Seventh and Fifth. Muma became close friends with one woman in particular. Dr. Barbara Richardson ran the emergency room of Mount Sinai Hospital, located a few blocks north of the meadow. Since the start of Jason's hospitalization, Muma had been consulting Barbara, who, in addition to managing the ER of a major hospital, had been bringing Muma food every week—steamed artichokes, lasagnas, pots of soup.

"Get him to Sinai," Barbara said early on.

We resisted her advice. We didn't want to move. Barbara said she had trained the head nurse of Mount Sinai's Neuro-ICU and vouched for her excellent work. Moreover, Mount Sinai was a bigger, stronger, newer facility than St. Vincent's.

"He's fine where he is," we said. Besides, Monica and I lived in Brooklyn, far from Mount Sinai. When Muma reported that Jason had fallen and then that the ventriculostomy had disconnected, Barbara again urged us to move. "We'll see," we said.

Then one day Jason's hands were different temperatures. "Right?" we said to the nurses, who agreed and wrapped Jason's cold left hand in a warm towel, an action that made me feel like we were not in New York City but in a primitive country with naive customs. The doctor of infectious disease was paged. Hours passed before she responded. Her conclusion: Jason's right hand, site of an earlier IV line, was infected. His left hand was not cold. His right hand was hot.

"I'm going to see if Sinai has a bed available," Barbara said.

Still we hesitated. Inertia had captured us. Fatigue was wearing us down. At least the problems at St. Vincent's were familiar. Was Mount Sinai a better hospital or a whole new round of trouble? What if moving him proved to be a mistake? We were clinging to the image of Jason recovering at St. Vincent's. To move to a second hospital was to kill this image. It was to acknowledge that the future was entirely unknown.

Two days later Jason was writhing in pain, unable to communicate.

"He's been doing that all morning," Bea said nonchalantly. And apparently during the night.

"I don't know," said the resident. "Other than the skin rash in his groin area."

They looked away, waiting for the problem to solve itself. The infectious disease doctor wasn't called. The pharmacy didn't respond. Bea refused to disengage Jason's catheter, saying she needed a doctor's order to do so. In periodic spurts Jason was grimacing, his body clenching, his breathing a series of short, shallow breaths. In a surreal way he looked like someone in labor.

"Does it feel like you need to pee?" Rop asked.

Jason managed to nod.

With Bea on her lunch break, the relief nurse recognized the severity of the situation. The catheter was blocked. Jason's bladder could burst. Not waiting for a doctor's approval, she removed the catheter. After taking a very long piss, Jason finally relaxed. And our inertia was finally broken.

"Where are we going?" asked Jason. He was lying in a stretcher wheeled by a nurse down one long hallway after another. Monica, Muma, and I trotted alongside him.

"To a different hospital," we said.

"How are we getting there?" he asked. Mute for days, he was suddenly loquacious.

"In an ambulance."

"Don't you think there's a more appropriate form of transportation?"

"Like what?" we said, laughing at the idea that there was anything more appropriate than an ambulance to transport a man unable to stand on his own, with a tube exiting his skull.

The move to Mount Sinai came quickly, factors suddenly in alignment. First, a bed opened up. Having always thought of hospitals as welcoming sanctuaries, I was startled to learn that often patients are turned away simply because all the beds are taken. Second, Jason's infection abruptly retreated. Hospitals don't like to take infected patients from other facilities because their current patients would be put at risk. So long as Jason's temperature and white blood cell count were elevated, he was stuck at St. Vincent's. But, as if on cue, his numbers had dropped to within a normal range.

Taking Jason and his discharge papers from the nurse, paramedics wheeled the stretcher across the Seventh Avenue sidewalk to a waiting ambulance. The late August sun shone sharply in the clear dry day.

"How does it feel to be outside?" I asked, aware that Jason hadn't breathed fresh air in twenty-six days.

"Disorienting," he said.

The fact that Jason had been born in Mount Sinai was not lost on me.

Would this be the story? To die where he was born.

The story about Jason's birth was that because Muma and Rop didn't have a bassinet, he came home in a cardboard box. The story about my birth was that the doctor, an opera buff, chatted up Rop about his days accompanying Leontyne Price and Jennie Tourel. "It's Brunhilde!" the doctor exclaimed when I emerged. The other story about my birth was that I was jaundiced and had to sleep in leg braces because my feet turned in. But at least I didn't come home in a cardboard box.

Barbara Richardson had run reconnaissance on which neuro-surgeon might be assigned to Jason. We wanted the chief, whom we saw as the big shot, the department's brand name, with the most experience under his belt. We thought "chief neurosurgeon" equaled "best neurosurgeon." But Jason was given to a doctor about whom Barbara could not tell us very much because he'd started working at Mount Sinai only a month before Jason's arrival.

Dr. Prithvi Narayan had become a neurosurgeon after a career as an electrical engineer, designing medical software for brain navigation. Yet he looked young. He was trim, with a buoyancy in his walk that told us that his not having a long neurosurgical career might be a bonus. Plus, we figured, being new, Dr. Narayan would need to prove himself. He might give Jason attention for which the chief didn't have the time or need. Dr. Narayan's serious, clear-eyed, compassionate demeanor seemed directly informed by a natural proclivity to understand how things worked.

In the waiting room outside the Neuro-ICU, Dr. Narayan said the most beautiful words I'd ever heard: "We're going to get Jason through this." The confidence in his voice was like the ocean's sandy floor touching the feet of the near-drowned. We had reached shore. We might still be lost, but at least we weren't going under.

After he left the waiting room, the four of us looked at each other, stunned and overjoyed. The doctor's words did not sound like a false promise. Rather, they indicated his intention to command the situation of which absent Dr. Glass had lost control—Dr. Glass, whose approach to medicine said, "First, accept defeat." Dr. Narayan was going to fight for Jason's life.

And yet wasn't that what doctors were supposed to do? Though relieved to be in Dr. Narayan's care—for he was, in many ways, treating not just Jason but all of us—I found it strange that we should see as fortune's gift this most basic aspect of the doctor's profession.

Our good luck was followed hard by bad. With Jason stable, his temperature normal and WBC down, Dr. Narayan had ordered an angiogram. An AVM had caused the bleed.

AVM: arteriovenous malformation, a tangle of blood vessels in which arteries run into veins without pressure-diffusing capillaries. Sometimes these blood vessels rupture.

The diagnosis brought some relief. We had an answer to the mystery. But it also brought dread. AVMs often rebleed. Jason's AVM was sitting on the top of his brain stem, the part of the brain controlling heartbeat and breathing.

Would this be the story? He lived a month, then the AVM bled again and he died.

I regretted every moment I'd relaxed in the past three and a half weeks. Dr. Glass's earliest warning, that Jason might not survive, echoed fresh in my mind. His life still hung precariously. He had survived one bleed. We could not assume he would survive another. We had been granted these three weeks—why, I could not say. Still, at any moment he might be taken from us.

Following the angiogram, Jason's condition plummeted. The infection from the disconnected ventriculostomy, which had abated, now exploded into meningitis, an inflammation of the meninges, the membranes surrounding the brain and spinal cord. The seizures returned, worse than before. He was in status epilepticus, a state in which his brain was stuck, one seizure following another. Jason looked like he was sleeping, but inside him an electrical storm was raging. He was running a fever. His white blood cell count was high. An X-ray showed fluid buildup in his lungs.

Dr. Narayan outlined his plan. Broad spectrum of antibiotics. Increased oxygen. New blood and urine analyses. MRI to look for abscesses (areas of infection that become walled off from the rest of the brain). Phenobarbital and Dilantin to break the seizures.

The word *phenobarbital* was like an artifact from my childhood, a cheap narrow paperback with a cover bent and torn at its corners, a grown-up's book whose dry brittle pages offered a glimpse of an era that by the mid-1970s was gone, though its conventions and language still hung in the air—the breakdowns and psych wards and lethargy-inducing medication of the 1950s and 1960s. And here was phenobarbital, decades later, keeping Jason's seizures at bay. I wasn't surprised that the drug had multiple uses, nor did its presence make me confuse Mount Sinai for a mental hospital. But its name laid bare that we were in deep waters.

There was another problem. Time had expired on the ventriculostomy. For nearly thirty days it had been moved, several times, across Jason's head and back. An internal shunt needed to be installed. Three weeks ago the idea of a shunt had repulsed us. We'd wanted Jason returned to his old unaltered self. Now everything except his survival fell away. A shunt? Do it. Just please, let him live.

"Nature has a good way of healing things," Dr. Narayan said after he'd presented his strategy. He always left room in the discussion for this aspect of Jason's recovery. In a major hospital, administering hardcore Western medicine, Dr. Narayan didn't forget about nature. Jason was young and strong. But I took the doctor's words to mean more than Jason's nature. They meant that

Mother Nature trended toward healing. Considering the calamities befalling Jason, it seemed radical to believe that the nature of Nature was to mend. But the idea felt comforting and true, and I wrote the doctor's words along the spine of my notebook, next to the outline of treatments and medications.

10

We were back in rough waters, no sight of shore.

A coma was induced. Slowing Jason's neurological activity would cut off the seizure cycle, probably. He was moved into the quarantine bay. Anyone seeing him, however briefly, put on gloves, gown, and mask. The nasogastric (nose-to-stomach) food tube, inserted during the seizures at St. Vincent's, was replaced with a percutaneous endoscopic gastronomy (PEG), which delivered food directly to his stomach. Instead of wearing an oxygen face mask, now he had a tracheotomy, an opening in his throat, which connected to a respirator.

"If there is a major problem," Dr. Narayan said, explaining the trach, "we don't want to be intubating him and dealing with the problem at the same time."

A major problem was a distinct possibility.

With heavy hearts we agreed to the trach and PEG, which so definitively marked Jason as a long-term patient. On the bright side, Dr. Narayan said, now Jason's face would be unobstructed. Many families found relief in that.

Seeing Jason's face gave us some comfort, but overall he did not look well. He had lost about fifty pounds—"I think he'd be happy to lose the first ten," Monica said—leaving his knees disproportionately large. Pillows between his knees and under his elbows provided some cushioning, but even the sheets were like sandpaper on his fragile skin. Open sores covered his back and heels. After losing fat, his body had started to drop muscle. Now only the most elemental muscle was left, muscle that lay closest to the bone. As if something were winching his body from within, his legs bent, his knuckles caved, his mouth was pulled into a fixed *O*. His feet were dropping. Confined to a bed, the human body falls apart with astonishing speed.

On Jason's third or fourth day at St. Vincent's, at the nurses' instruction, Rop had bought a pair of high-top sneakers to help Jason's feet maintain a right angle to his legs. Now we were shown how to put on and take off—don and doff, in hospital parlance— puffy blue foot braces. Nurses taught us how to shift Jason from one side to the other. Like clockwork, we turned him.

Rop brought his electric razor and shaved Jason's face. Monica clipped and filed his nails. We cleaned his mouth, learning from nurses how to swab and suction the mucus and gunk. We were scrambling to protect Jason's humanness. Already his smell had changed to the pseudo-sweet chemical smell of a body saturated with drugs and sustained by formulated food, a body whose breath drew on the calibrated air of a respirator, a body washed with disposable cloths that came in individual plastic packets that were heated in a microwave.

One night, leaving, I paused, watching Jason and the numbers on the monitor beside him. He lay on his back, his lungs rhythmically rising with air pumped in from the respirator. His body looked mostly gone. But his heart was pounding a tough steady beat. This man has a strong constitution, I thought. I remembered the time he walloped a cab driver who had threatened Muma, the time he lambasted hecklers at a show, the time he jumped in a lake and rescued our drowning cousin. His booming heart said I fight. I fight. I fight.

The bed rails were like a barricade between Jason and the rest of the world. I didn't speak the official language of his medical condition, but my gut said that if a person didn't touch or smell or hear familiar people, his brain would fall apart. Consciously, I put myself on his side, resting my hand on him, adjusting his sheets and pillows and bolsters, holding his hand in mine like we were shaking on a deal. And even though he had tubes going in and out all over, I embraced him—gently, carefully, wrapping my arms around his bony shoulders.

The nurses told us to tape pictures to the walls so that when Jason opened his eyes he would see familiar faces. Read to him, said the nurses. Play music. Hug him. Talk to him. Assume he can hear you. Picture him walking, talking, playing the guitar. Ask him to picture walking, talking, and playing the guitar too. At St. Vincent's our efforts to engage Jason had been met with tolerant indifference, but at Mount Sinai these efforts were encouraged and expanded. It was a relief to stop feeling like the eccentric family.

Rop read him the *Times*. I read short stories by Philip K. Dick, to whom Jason had introduced me with *Do Androids Dream of Electric Sheep?* The tales of questionable realities, alternate universes, and elaborate dream states seemed exceptionally appropriate. If Jason was processing his circumstances, perhaps he could imagine himself the hero of a science fiction story.

The bay filled with big color photographs of friends and family as well as Jason and Monica's cats, Rudy and Mario. The nurses said we should hang pictures so Jason would see familiar faces, but these pictures had an effect on us too. Here was Jason outside a club, kneeling with his arms outstretched, in front of a group of musicians, the picture capturing a moment of silly exuberance. In another Jason stood proudly next to Rop's ninety-nine-year-old mother, Boo. Another picture showed Jason onstage, playing guitar, his slack face and half-closed eyes testifying to his deep absorption in the music. Another: Jason and Monica, close-up in black-and-white, the picture taken in a photo booth at a wedding reception, their faces reflecting love and the small details—Monica's pearl

49

earrings, Jason's smart suit—reminders of the glamorous evening. Each picture provoked a memory that Monica, Muma, Rop, and I shared while sitting around silent sleeping Jason. The mood was not funereal. We were still prone to sidesplitting laughter, and more than once the nurses asked us to keep it down. But just as mourners feel the presence of the deceased as they swap stories, so we summoned Jason.

Along with dozens of cards and letters, a stuffed German shepherd from Sandy Bell, and a gourd piano, a growing pile of CDs crowded the night table cabinet. Some were mixes sent by friends. Some were albums on which Jason played that had been released while he was in the hospital. Some were albums we brought in, carefully choosing music we knew Jason preferred, such as traditional Indian music and American blues. I couldn't imagine a worse purgatory for a musician than being forced to listen to music he didn't like. And we played live comedy albums by Steve Martin and Bill Cosby, the sound of jokes and applause filling Jason's quarantine bay while we sat beside him, terrified.

September 14. I wonder how it is for Jason, floating in the netherworld, asleep asleep asleep. Darkness—or dreams?

The world seemed made of glass, sharp and easily broken. I moved through it ever surprised at the solidity of objects, expecting walls to shatter when I brushed against them. Columbia Prep had given Muma a semester's leave, but I returned to my secretarial job, where on slow days I sat at my desk, simply feeling the chair beneath me and the table under my elbows. In those moments sorrow covered me like snow on a statue.

Part of my mind stopped, but another part moved frantically on. I read articles about AVMs, researched surgery options, skimmed online support group postings—searching for Jason's story with the right ending. I found endings that were happy, sad, and everything in between. The archetypal brain hemorrhage didn't exist.

At the hospital one thought chased another. Should we stretch Jason's arms and legs and fingers? Clean his mouth? When was he last turned to a different side? Should we play music? A different album? Read a story? Some time between getting on the subway at Ninety-Sixth and Lexington and getting off at Fifteenth and Prospect Park West, I switched back to spacing out. But I was always carrying around my other self, the manic on overdrive or the slumberer half-dead to the world.

The scope of my life shrank to work, hospital, home. The hospital was where I felt alive and normal. Otherwise, I didn't want to be around people, I didn't want to go out, I didn't want to think.

Sometimes I felt tested—by what, I didn't know—to see if I would speak one way to Jason and another to friends. But I never did. I thought of athletes preparing for competition who would not tolerate any possibility but winning. Of course, some of them lost. But until the final bell, they remained absolutely devoted to victory.

Often I exhaled only after realizing that I had been holding my breath for an extended period of time.

The coma broke Jason's seizures. But he contracted pneumonia. An infection led to the removal of the prized shunt, replaced by another ventriculostomy. His liver and appendix were suffering from the heavy drugs in his system. The NG feeding tube, replaced by the stomach PEG, had left a problem in his sinuses. His temperature was rarely normal, though it was unclear whether that was in response to an infection or if his brain's thermostat had been damaged. His lungs almost collapsed when air was caught under his rib cage. Barely had one urinary tract infection ended before another began. And he was not waking up.

At Dr. Narayan's suggestion we scheduled a meeting with the chief of neurosurgery. Afraid the AVM would rebleed, we wanted to discuss Jason's options. In my notebook I dutifully wrote a list of our questions. What kind of surgery should we consider? What are the risks? What is the most common outcome? How many have you performed? What is the chance of rebleed over time? Crowded into the chief's cramped office, we started through our list of questions. The chief gave us some answers. The brain needed six to twelve weeks to absorb the blood. The rebleed risk was cumulative, as high as 6 percent the first year. Smaller AVMs had a higher risk of rebleed. Jason's AVM was small.

But he didn't want to talk about surgery. "We view Jason's case as very grave," he said. In other words, it wasn't worth discussing treatment for the AVM because Jason probably wasn't going to survive.

I heard nothing after that. With friends and colleagues I always framed the conversation in affirmative terms. The most defeatist words I allowed myself to say were "I don't know." And here we'd come to the expert, to the chief, wanting to discuss the future, asking his professional opinion. With a single sentence he'd rendered irrelevant our long list of questions. In his eyes Jason was so close to death that his life wasn't worth consideration.

"That was awful," I said, as we waited for the elevator afterward. "How do you guys feel?"

"Defiant," Muma replied.

Monica and Rop immediately heartily agreed, and their conviction drowned my fear.

I would be defiant too.

September 20. I dreamed I was in bed with him. He was naked and had no tubes attached to him. He wasn't speaking, he was silent—muted. But his eyes were telling me something. He was telling me something with his eyes as he embraced me.

One night, when Monica was staying at a friend's apartment in Manhattan, I stopped by their place to feed Rudy and Mario. After putting out food and fresh water for the cats, I stepped into Jason's studio. Everything was exactly as he had left it when he'd walked out the door on August 4. Instruments and equipment surrounded his desk, which was littered with picks, guitar strings, a metronome, composition notebooks, and pages of scribbled lyrics to songs he was writing or learning. As if examining a painting ripped in half, I felt the break in his life.

Monica's decision to move was no surprise. "It's too hard to live among Jason's absence," she said. Four months pregnant, she was commuting from home in Brooklyn to work in Manhattan, then farther uptown to the hospital in Spanish Harlem, before going back to Brooklyn after visitors' hours ended, arriving home at ten at night or later.

I worried what Jason would think about a new apartment. But Monica said neither of them had liked the old place. One night, she said, as they were going out, they saw a man across the street pissing on a building. "Jason's face clouded over," she said. "He hated living in a neighborhood where people did things like that."

She found a place on Ninety-Fifth Street, a short walk from Mount Sinai. The weekend of the move, dozens of friends showed up to pack boxes, wrangle the cats, load the truck, unload the truck, unpack boxes, put dishes in cabinets, set up the stereo, move furniture, hang clothes in the closet.

These friends helped again when Rachel Loshak organized a concert at the Living Room to raise money for medical and living expenses. A singer and bassist, Rachel wrote sharply beautiful songs, and Jason had not only played with her for many years but had contributed significantly to her particular sound. Some shows were just the two of them, but the music was full and complex, with her bass, his guitar, her clear soprano voice. The sold-out benefit raised twenty thousand dollars.

At the request of Monica, Muma, and Rop, I said a few words of thanks on behalf of the family. Onstage I felt fine, but later, when I saw a photograph, I recognized the look in my eyes as pure fear.

October 1. R, a fellow patient from St. Vincent's, found Jay at Mount Sinai. R was walking into walls. The general practitioner said, It's stress. R continued to walk into walls. The eye doctor said, I don't see a problem, but if you were my son, I'd send you to a neurologist. The neurologist ordered an MRI. The insurance agency wouldn't cover an MRI with dye without cause. When R came out of the MRI, the technicians said, Hold on, we're putting you back in with dye. Insurance needs cause, R protested. Oh, there's cause, they said but wouldn't tell him what it was. With an appointment with the neurologist scheduled for the next morning, he couldn't wait. He tracked the doctor down. A tumor the size of a lemon. They got it out.

Jason opened his eyes but remained uncommunicative and unresponsive. A nurse saw him move a leg. A nurse saw him move his arm. These rare slight actions were momentous, but we knew how quickly the trapdoor could fall open. To see him yawn was a triumph, but joy took its place next to unrelenting dread.

"We don't know how much patients understand in that twilight zone," Barbara Richardson said. How rare to hear a doctor say "We don't know." And how comforting. I didn't want closure. I didn't want a prognosis. I wanted *anything's possible.* Not only should we be reading, playing music, talking to him, talking about him, hugging him, grooming him, but we should keep our minds open for other ways we might engage him. *We don't know* what will work, but doing nothing could mean wasting a crucial opportunity.

Wondering what might reach a person in this twilight zone, I recalled the summer of 1997, when Jason spent three months in an ashram in India, where he meditated for hours every day, guided by the ashram's founder, Osho, through recordings made before he died. Perhaps the soft timbre and slow cadence of Osho's voice could hook Jason's mind. From Osho's website I downloaded a lecture, "From Unconsciousness to Consciousness."

"Jay," I said. Lying in bed, eyes closed, he made no response. "I'm going to play a recording of a talk given by Osho."

At the sound of the guru's name, Jason's eyebrows shot up. His eyes did not open, but everything about his expression said, "Oh, really?" He had heard me.

Like this, he would appear. Nothing for hours or days, then a fleeting but clear expression on his face, a single definitive squeeze in his handshake. He was there, buried deep, but he was there.

11

"Hello, Jason," Dr. Narayan would say in his strong voice. "Jason, shake my hand."

Dr. Narayan possessed a magnetism that seemed absolutely right for his profession, confidence mixed with unvarnished kindness. With Dr. Narayan there was no playing up his neurosurgeon status. He did not surround himself with interns and residents but strode into Jason's bay, his white coat billowing behind him, many times each day, to talk to us, to talk to Jason. He believed, as we did, that Jason could recover. "I will have him back to enjoy your baby," he said to Monica, and because Dr. Narayan had two little girls, we felt this could not be an idle pledge.

Such was our relationship with Dr. Narayan that it did not seem odd when he told us he'd enlisted his mother-in-law to pray for Jason, and in turn she had asked her entire town in India to pray for Jason too. One of the nurses told us that she had been planning to become an actress until she had a calling from God to go into medicine. We took these stories as omens and held onto them fiercely. Muma consulted a Buddhist lama, who recommended "kindness to animals." A viral email requesting the same of family and friends led to several adoptions of stray cats and dogs. Before seeing Jason, I knelt in the hospital's nondenominational chapel. Day after day I wrote in the prayer book, "Please watch over my brother."

I didn't think written prayers were more effective than spoken ones, but I was drawn to this collection of requests and gratitudes. Some of the entries gave specifics—name, room number, illness. Some were lengthy. Some were illegible, in a different language or in handwriting that curled and overlapped so much it blocked itself out. I put down the same five words every time. The act gave me a modest satisfaction. In the future someone could look through the book and find this record of my devotion.

I had learned to pray for real when I got sober. *Help*, in the morning. *Thanks*, at night. Sobriety was the first time, as an adult, that I had considered whether I believed in God. Muma and Rop had never taken Jason and me to church. Both had been raised in oppressive organized religion and wanted nothing more to do with it. But after going to a Christian horseback riding summer camp, I constructed a chapel in the woods behind our house and delivered a sermon plagiarized from the camp's pastor, "Are You a Champ or a Chump?" Cast as the Virgin Mary in the school Christmas pageant, I understood the assignment to be divinely given and, long after the pageant had ended, continued to raise and lower my hands over Baby Jesus, who was usually manifesting as an ear of dried corn.

Sometimes while Muma and Rop played shows, Jason and I spent the afternoon and evening with a family whose two oldest daughters matched us in age. Their mother was born-again. Their father was an atheist who said, "After you die, the worms eat you, and that's it." Following dinner, which included goat's milk fresh from their farm, the mother read and talked about the Bible. She gave us soft thin pamphlets of illustrated parables, accompanied by paper dolls. This was called Devotion, and as it consisted of books and dolls, I loved it. After saying our prayers aloud, the two oldest daughters and Jason and I would lay our sleeping bags around a campfire in the backyard and stay up late telling ghost stories. My experience of their religion was inextricable from the mother's gentle voice, the beautiful log house they'd built with their own hands, their horses and pigs and the goat that butted me in the back one sad afternoon, fast rides on the father's motorcycle, the dog who was named after the mother's first husband (who had died at sea), their long driveway through the woods, and the Airstream trailer parked there in which the oldest daughter had been born.

In my twenties I started meditating, attending weekly dharma discourses in New York and retreats at Buddhist monasteries. I was attracted to the idea of stopping my mind from thinking—or at least trying to. All of my education, from secondary school through college, had been based on intellectual rhetoric. But my questions and concerns—Why do I feel such despair? Leave New York, or will moving solve nothing?—were impervious to logic and reason. Everything is as it should be, says Buddhism. For a long time I felt the truth of this precept while simultaneously rejecting it completely. How could everything be as it should when I didn't have so many things that I wanted?

Once I found myself walking up Fourth Avenue next to a Buddhist monk. I greeted him. He said hello.

"Where do you practice?" I asked.

He smiled. "Everywhere." Then, after a beat, he added, "Thirty-Third and Sixth," and handed me a business card.

Meditation was what had helped me realize that I needed to get sober. When I'd started drinking and smoking herb, I had an overwhelming desire for experience. For a while I had a great ride. Music was more intense, jokes were funnier, everything felt cool. Then the fun ran out. That which I had been chasing had totally escaped my grasp. Even as my writing was beginning to be produced and published, a nagging fear grew inside me that I wasn't a writer but a lush, and I wanted to write more than I wanted any cocktail or joint. So I quit.

Being sober was the first time as an adult that I contemplated whether a divine power existed. I let go of what I'd absorbed as a child and what I thought society wanted me to believe. "Do I see God in the mountains, the moon, a blade of grass, a baby's smile, anyone's smile?" I wrote at the time. "Yes, and I see these things as they are."

My vision of God was math and science as well as poetry and dance. Not an old bearded man—God didn't "want" anything. Rather, I saw God as a process, an awakening. At the same time, I prayed to God, morning and night, and it didn't matter then what I envisioned because it was not God but the action itself, kneeling and praying, that gave me faith.

After Jason's hemorrhage I prayed in the morning, I prayed at night, I prayed in the private bathroom at work, I prayed in the hospital's chapel. The meat of my message remained the same: Jason is alive. Thank you. Please help us get through today.

In praying, I was promising to do everything I could while recognizing that part of Jason's recovery lay beyond human power. The best medicine and our greatest efforts might not suffice. Would fate be cruel or kind? I disregarded this question. I could not make demands.

Whatever happened, I wanted no regrets. I could think of people whose friendship I'd spurned, opportunities I'd arrogantly rejected, words I'd said that I would pay money to take back. Not this. I needed to know that I had done everything I could. Only then would I be able to accept whatever the future turned out to be.

October 20. What is it to lie mute and entirely at the mercy of others? Sometimes I am overwhelmed with sadness. Jason? The goodest guy in the universe.

On October 21 Jason left the Neuro-ICU. He had survived a brain hemorrhage, meningitis, seizures, a coma, pneumonia, a half-dozen surgeries (including an appendectomy), and what felt like a thousand infections.

Before entering rehabilitation, he needed to be weaned off the respirator. Patients on respirators become dependent on them, so the machines can't be disconnected abruptly. The area of the brain that oversees breathing—recognizes the necessity and commands the physical action—realizes that oxygen is coming in on a regular basis and stops working. I had been relieved, as Jason's condition worsened, to see the steady rise and fall of his chest as the machine piped in good air. In the Respiratory Intensive Care Unit (RICU: the "rick-you") the respirator would be turned off, first for short periods of time, then longer and longer, until Jason started to inhale and exhale on his own again.

It was a strange paradox that in order to save Jason's brain, we had intentionally done something to debilitate it. For the greater purpose of his recovery we had compromised his ability to breathe. The reasoning made sense—if in an unexpected crisis Jason's lungs collapsed and he wasn't on the respirator, he might die—but I marveled at how easily the brain could be duped. In parts no longer active, it atrophied. The brain needed *need*.

At last we were not going to the Neuro-ICU. We were not putting on protective gowns and gloves. We went to a different floor in a different unit of the hospital. In the eerily calm RICU time seemed to have stopped. The patients, who came from all over the hospital, were concentrating on the same single feat: taking a breath.

Long gone were our expectations that Jason's hospitalization would end quickly. Even as we rejoiced to leave the Neuro-ICU, we turned to the next stage of our terrible adventure with exhaustion and apprehension. Would his next doctor and nurses be as dedicated as Dr. Narayan and the nurses in the Neuro-ICU?

And yet if Jason were to recover and come home, we would have to take this step. I realized then that we—Muma, Rop, Monica, myself—would go with him from hospital to hospital, from unit to unit, in a way that no doctor could match. There would be no single savior—deep down I still wanted a savior—but, rather, different people along the way, assigned by fate. Jason was less dependent on a person than on the luck of the draw, which doctor's name came up upon his admittance.

Please, please, I prayed. Give him another Narayan.

We continued to read to him, play music, massage him, clean his mouth, talk to him, cut his nails, shave his face. Every day his ventilator was turned off for a period of time and every day he breathed a little longer on his own.

November 10. The woman in the next-door bed is not long for this world, in a coma, her liver shut down, her stomach rejecting food. Her son, an NYPD officer, is there nightly. I try to be still so he can have the space. Tonight he leaned over her, sobbing. "You'll be in the Lord's hands. Everything's going to be okay. You know that, right, Ma?" He must have said "I love you" a hundred times.

November 11. A dream last night. Jay was talking. Nothing special, just normal. I looked up at him—he was giant—with such awe that Monica and Muma and Rop laughed at me. I was incredulous at the (his) human spirit and ability to endure.

November 12. This morning the woman's family came to the hospital and gathered around the matriarch. A minister delivered the last rites and turned off the respirator. A little while later she died. By evening her bed was remade and clean, as were the walls—stripped of the Halloween card, the picture of schoolchildren with Spiderman, the postcard invitation from Columbia University to something that has happened by now. Even the telephone was gone. The area was as blank as a hotel room between checked-in guests.

The woman was old. She was expected to die. Still, bearing witness to the end of her life reminded me how close Jason was. Death was in the next bed over.

12

Another dream: I enter Jason's room but he is gone. His bed is empty. He's not dead, just somewhere else. He's missing.

On November 16 I came to the RICU after work, as always feeling late, wanting to have been there all day instead of arriving when the sky was dark, the night shift on. As in my dream, his bed was empty. All mention of him had disappeared. For a moment my mind was suspended. He can't be dead, he's dead, where was the phone call?

"He's gone to Rehabilitation," said the soft-spoken nurse who had taken care of him. She gave me directions. Rehab was in another building.

"It was a pleasure," she said when I thanked her. "Especially for him."

"He's special," I said, and both of us started to cry. I felt like our ship was pulling out of port and I was waving at the nurse back on shore.

"Bring him back to say hi sometime," she said, adding emphatically, "Walking."

November 16. First eleventh floor. Then eighth floor. Then ninth floor. Now third floor.

Mount Sinai spread over several blocks, a patchwork of buildings added over the past century. A modern black skyscraper with a glass-walled lobby housed the Neuro-ICU and the RICU, but Rehab was in a low white-brick building designed in the utilitarian style of the 1960s. The sweaty-sock smell of unwell bodies filled its harsh bright halls. Everything was beige or gray. I found Jason in room 303, where some of the vertical window blinds were missing. Those remaining drew open only halfway. The window, right above the building's blue awning entrance, faced a playground in the George Washington Carver projects on the far side of Madison Avenue.

The move was abrupt but not unexpected. Once Jason had started to breathe on his own, insurance—that is, his private health insurance—had begun to question whether he needed to be in the Respiratory ICU. He may have been too well for the RICU, but he was not ready for Rehab.

He slept as if under a spell. After the chaos of the Neuro-ICU, sleep had felt right, a relief. But now, three and a half weeks later, his sleep raised questions. Was his body restoring itself? Or was he having seizures? Or was he knocked out by the (umpteenth) urinary tract infection, not a big deal for a healthy person but potentially destructive for someone as vulnerable as Jason? Or was he too sedated by phenobarbital, the antiseizure medication? A precautionary EEG noncommittally reported "activity" in his brain. Like chatter on the terrorist airwaves, it would prove meaningful only after something awful happened.

Having shared a bedroom with him for fourteen years, I knew how he slept—hot, heavy, a snorer who could, to my envy, wake up for the earliest Saturday morning cartoons. In the night I would push him onto his side or shake him. "Stop snoring!" "Sorry," he would sigh, still asleep. Once a bat flew into the bedroom that the four of us were sharing, temporarily, in one of Goodspeed's houses for actors. Muma screamed and ducked under the covers,

Rop chased it with a broom, I sang the *Batman* theme song, and Jason slept.

After the multipronged assault on his brain and the deterioration of his body, after the infections and coma, after the medications to fight the infections and induce the coma—and given that his natural sleep resembled hibernation—asking Jason to participate in speech or physical therapy was like asking him to swim from the bottom of the ocean to its surface while carrying an anchor.

The neurologist—I'll call her Dr. Dear—refused to consider changing the phenobarbital dose. Despite a reputation as "New York's best," Dr. Dear had the bedside manner of gravel. "I don't know how you're getting through this," she said to Monica, and when Muma excitedly reported that Jason had moved a finger on command, Dr. Dear gave her a long stony stare while slowly shaking her head.

His sluggishness was due to the seizures, said Dr. Dear, and too bad, we would have to put up with phenobarbital's sedative effects for the rest of his life because another seizure could cause permanent brain damage. Her tone of voice implied that disagreeing with her meant we *wanted* Jason to have permanent brain damage.

Monica had fought with insurance for Jason to stay in the RICU until he woke up, at least until the UTI cleared. Wising up to the company's tactics, we could see that if Jason were unable to participate in Rehab's therapies, insurance would expel him using the same logic by which it had moved him out of the RICU, that is, by saying it was not *suitable* for him to be there. If insurance forced him out of Rehab, then what? We had no idea.

In fact, by this point—mid-November, about three months after the initial bleed—Jason's coverage was on the brink of hitting its million-dollar limit, although no one knew it at the time—not Mount Sinai; not Monica; not her father, Lou, or stepmother, Jane, both of whom were helping track the bills. Even the insurance company didn't know. The tally didn't exist in real time, partly because the insurance company maintained a policy that if it didn't receive a bill by a certain date following treatment, it would not pay for the treatment. Mount Sinai didn't bill anywhere close to this deadline, meaning that invoices were circling from Mount Sinai to insurance back to Mount Sinai to Monica, whose phone calls to Eileen, the insurance rep, were, Monica said, "like talking to a wall."

November 16. As in the RICU, there is a sign recommending that patients make arrangements to leave before 10 a.m. on the day of their discharge. As before, I read the sign quizzically—checking out has been a faraway event. Now, though, it feels like this could be the place where that happens.

The move to Rehab had been rushed, inelegant, unnatural. Still, we forced ourselves to focus on the bright side. Jason was no longer in an intensive care unit of any kind. The days since August 4 had been an arduous detour, but we were back on track. We saw Rehab as the place where the magic happened, the last stop before home.

In leaving the RICU, Jason moved out of Dr. Narayan's purview. He didn't need a neurosurgeon now but a physiatrist, a doctor of rehabilitation. I'll call him Dr. Rooney, because while walking down Fifty-Eighth Street the same week Jason moved to Rehab, I passed by Andy Rooney, the *60 Minutes* commentator. "Can I take your picture?" I said, to which the famous curmudgeon barked, "No!"

Mild-mannered Dr. Rooney set Tuesdays at 4:00 as a regular time for Muma, Rop, Monica, and me to meet with him and the social worker, who looked about twenty years old. Having a scheduled time for conversation pleased and reassured us. We saw it as the type of deliberate, organized action that would be made by a doctor capable of returning Jason to health. Moreover, to our great relief, Dr. Rooney agreed that Jason should get off phenobarbital. The EEG indicated no brain damage from the seizures, he said, and he promised to talk to Dr. Dear about lowering the dose.

In the family lounge, a perpetually empty afterthought of a room with a view of an alley, we reunited with the Italian family we had met in the Neuro-ICU. Their patient was a man near Jason's age, married, with a young child. His mother was living at Mount Sinai, sleeping in the lounge, washing her clothes in the coin-op laundry room.

"After the wash, just put your bra on—it dries in an hour," she told Muma and me, as if we were neighbors trading housekeeping tips instead of families encamped in a hospital.

The physical therapists dressed Jason in a T-shirt and sweatpants and helped him sit on the side of the bed, though they didn't *help* him so much as *put* him there, for he had absolutely no strength, no ability to move any part of his body. Unlike when he sat in the chair at St. Vincent's, the moment was marked not by triumph but agony. His emaciated body looked like it had been crumpled up into a ball and was unfurling feebly, almost against its own will. His head slumped forward, too heavy to hold up. His back was a semi-circle. With his eyelids half-closed, he seemed like a child roused in the middle of the night, in the middle of deep sleep, except he was not a child but a man and he appeared to be not 34 years old but 134. His glasses, too loose on his gaunt face, slid to the tip of his nose. His mouth hung open, pulled by contracted muscles in his face and jaw. A line of drool fell from his bottom lip. The tracheotomy remained in his throat, a short embedded pipe whose open end symbolized Jason's overall vulnerability.

Watching him, I felt like someone was stomping on my heart.

Give it a week, I thought. The situation will look so different.

I was alluding to summer camp, where the first week always lasted a year, then all the rest happened in a microsecond. But that first week was brutal, conjuring my days in the Sixty-Third Street Y nursery school, where, when I couldn't curl up in the reading loft, I would hide from my roughhousing classmates by sliding inside my cubby. I was shy, cowed, though I learned to mask this reality behind a joker's persona. In sixth grade I crowned myself class clown. From adolescence on, many of my decisions, big and small, were attempts to purge, avoid, overcome, or somehow dodge this fragility, clawing my way into A-level classes, performing in plays, spending three summers at Interlochen, a summer camp for the arts—three wretched first weeks—which was ultimately amazing but also cutthroat competitive. None of these things made me feel less frangible. So I would make myself remember this: in my first week at my first camp—Camp Kahdalea, when I was nine—I cried every night. A month later, as we stood around the lake, holding candles, singing "Barges," I cried again, and Jane Lyle Culpepper consoled me, saying, "Don't cry, Mojie. Tomorrow you're going home."

"I don't want to go home," I replied. "I don't want it to end."

In Jason's first days in Rehab my throat closed and my chest clenched, and dominating every moment was the desire to go home, to go back to when Jason's injury hadn't happened, an insatiable desire that I could only tuck into a recess of my heart. It rode with me everywhere, its presence evident some times more than others, never totally forgotten.

In the beginning Jason's inertia left the therapists with little to do. The physical therapist stretched him and taught us the stretches. Evenings we pushed and pulled his arms and legs and face and fingers and toes, which, like our old Plastic Man action figure, elongated but always returned to the shape of the mold.

Physical therapy would help him move. Speech therapy would help him talk. But what was occupational therapy? Was its purpose to refashion Jason's career according to his limited abilities? Simple repetitive activities came to mind—stamping expiration dates on canned fish.

Like the other therapists, the OT was athletic, trim, and young—too young, I worried, to have experience in the field, beyond the books.

Occupational therapy, she explained, started with daily activities like washing, dressing, "grooming."

She put a hairbrush in Jason's hand and guided his arm to the top of his head. I didn't understand. Did Jason usually brush his hair? Or did he comb it? Or did he use his fingers? And wouldn't he be able to do this if only he were more awake? I said nothing, but the exercise felt strange, false, as if she were asking Jason to play make-believe.

November 21. He was awake and alert though not responsive. Trapped inside? Paralyzed? Patience. Patience.

The speech therapist suggested that we find a nonvocal way for Jason to indicate yes and no. Could he put his thumb up and down? Could he raise one finger versus two? What set of contrasting movements could he make, reliably? "Close your eyes if—," we said. If you're in pain. If you want to turn over. Our binary code had the single signal—a blink—and its absence. We posed a question, and if he did nothing, we rephrased the question in its reverse. Close your eyes if you're okay. Close you're eyes if you're not okay. From there we would grope toward whatever he was trying to express. Close your eyes if your legs hurt. Close your eyes if you want to listen to another album.

Establishing two-way communication, limited as it was, was a huge step forward, for we had been relying on signs: was he sweaty? unusually tight? wild-eyed? what was his pulse? Records of his heartbeat filled my journal like weather reports. "Pulse high but got down in the 80s." "Pulse in the 120s & 130s, about 118 when I left." "Now sleeping, pulse 90." His pulse was his tempo, his telegraph, the Morse code of his inner state.

We talked to him, but what we said could not have lasted in his mind longer than the time our words spent in the air between us. It mattered that he heard our voices and knew we were there, but music was a better messenger. When we played Shuggie Otis or

Brij Bhushan Kabra, Jason wore his usual music listening expression: absorbed and engaged.

One night his pulse was at 125 beats per minute. In the hospital Jason's pulse was often higher than the standard healthy range of 60–100, but 125 was very high, evidence of distress. "Close your eyes if—." We tried every scenario, but he was too far in to respond. Rop and I shifted him to his left side, his right side. We stretched his arms, his legs. Monica cleaned his mouth. For thirty minutes we searched for the problem. Then, by chance, Monica put on a Beatles album, and Jason's pulse steadily began to come down.

At last Dr. Dear responded to Dr. Rooney's question: she would not take Jason off phenobarbital. She would not even bring down the dose.

If we asked for a different neurologist—if we fired "New York's best"—would we gain a reputation as a difficult, finicky family?

On phenobarbital he would never have another seizure, but how much speech and thought and movement would he recover?

Off phenobarbital he had a better chance of regaining his mind and body, but more seizures could harm him irrevocably.

We asked that Dr. Dear be replaced with a neurologist who would lower the dose. When I imagined explaining the decision to Jason, I found myself saying, We took the risk. We saw no other way for you to make it back.

13

Friday nights, leaving the hospital, I walked to the 107th Street garage where Muma parked her car, which I kept on weekends so that I could arrive at the start of visitors' hours, giving her and Rop a break from early mornings. And so that on Saturday afternoons I could drive with Lila to the beach at Riis Park in Far Rockaway.

Abandoned on the street, Lila had been taken in by a dog walker who'd put up a FOUND DOG sign, which I saw coming home one warm fall night and read as, *you* FOUND *your* DOG. When Lila felt safe, she was so sweet "it breaks your heart," as Muma once said. But threatened or startled, she could be ferocious. A man stopped us once, saying, "I know that dog. She bites." "She never bit me," I replied. But I saw more than a few squirrels breathe their last between her teeth, and she'd fight with other dogs. Walking in Prospect Park, she usually stayed on the leash.

On the empty beach she cut loose, flying across the sand, free. Part greyhound, she could move. Most days I felt closed in, restrained, but to see Lila run, to look out at the wide ocean, to have so much space to ourselves, to walk and walk and not on cement, I opened up. A cluster of colorful cabanas, relics of another era, was our turnaround point. Or we wandered through the dunes around the cannon at Fort Tilden.

I could take care of Lila. I could help at the hospital. I could show up for work. I couldn't do more. Inertia pushed at me like the wind on the beach. The soreness in my neck and shoulders and feet was unrelenting. There was never enough sleep. Laundry piled up. The apartment went uncleaned. Rewrites were due on my play, which was being produced by Carnegie Mellon in March. *Rewrites*, read the top of my to-do list, carried over from list to list.

November 21. It was very hard to walk into Jason's room this morning. Alone he slept in his wheelchair in a contorted position. I had to shake myself and say, Buck up. Strong face! Come on! I got through it.

This was Jason. This solitude, this silence, the prison of his body, the distance to his mind. Adrift on a lifeboat in the most remote sea.

In a breath I swapped my emotions so the person greeting him was ready and helpful, a representative from a benevolent world.

My guess was he couldn't grasp the big picture. As much as he was aware, it was an unreliable present-moment awareness. If in that present moment he detected that I was devastated, horrified, angry—what effect would that have? Might he think he'd caused those feelings? Better to focus on my relief that he was alive, move him to a more comfortable position, clean the drool, put on music, say hello knowing I was greeting the same Jason I had greeted all my life. I could be with him, a neutral normal thing, like the sunlight, like the children's shouts from the playground across the street.

Lila had accustomed me to shredded closet doors, chewed-up cardboard boxes, feathers and pieces of pillow covering the floor. Don't react to the destruction, I was advised by the patient men and women who taught our many obedience training classes. Ignore the bad and praise her when she's good, I was told. So I had some practice of walking into an upsetting scene and saying only, "Oh," and finding a way, against my first instinct, to act unperturbed. I could concentrate on what Jason had, not on what he lacked. Stay neutral or celebrate his progress, no matter how minute.

The sight of him those mornings showed clearly what his unimpeded course would be.

I believed he could recover.

I had to fight to give that hope its due chance.

November 25. Sometimes you have to sign the Waiver of Assumptions, which reads, I acknowledge that, for better or worse, anything can be, and anything can happen.

The Neuro-ICU had saved Jason's life. The RICU had helped him breathe on his own. In Rehab the goal was unclear. Sometimes I thought the therapists were just killing time. But what did I know? Maybe this was how a person recovered from a bleed in his head.

"Jason!" the PT said in a loud voice. She was holding a basket filled with toy fruit. "Can you *pick* the *banana* from the basket of *apples?* Pick the *banana.*"

I wouldn't care about a plastic banana either.

Slowly, excruciatingly slowly, he picked the banana.

The therapists were hampered by the New York nurses' union, which required that only nurses and nurse's aides attend to a patient's toileting needs, so when Jason was in the gym during a PT session and his catheter leaked or he defecated, the therapist would bring him back to his room. By the time someone came, fixed his catheter, cleaned him, and changed him into fresh clothes, his hour for therapy would be over, often the only hour of the day in which he exercised or even left his room.

November 28. When I arrived, the nurses were getting him into the wheelchair. It took a while. It's infuriating and defeating when they treat him like an object, a thing to be cleaned, dressed, moved, as opposed to a person who can hear and see, even if he can't walk and talk.

Most of the nurses were kind and professional. A few were paragons. In any other place we could have shrugged off the insensitive comments, like the condescending lecture Muma received while massaging Jason's feet.

"I wouldn't do that if I were you," a nurse said, sounding like the villain in a melodrama. I could feel my mother's agony. The nurse's tone of voice obscured her valid explanation—a massage could move a blood clot in Jason's foot to his heart or lungs or brain. As if to prove her knowledge, the nurse told us about her son, who had a traumatic brain injury from a car accident.

We did not say that perhaps the nurse should be working in a different unit. We did not say that her disapproval seemed colored by her personal situation. We said nothing. We let ourselves be her punching bag.

Mornings he was sweaty and excessively tense—what was happening when we weren't there?—so, using donations from relatives, we hired nurses from a private agency to sit with him through the night.

"He won't remember any of this," Dr. Rooney said.

"So he won't remember how devoted we were?" Muma asked with a laugh.

"I'll tell him," Dr. Rooney said. "I promise."

The nurses, the therapists, room 303, the gym at the end of the hall—would all fall away.

But would he have a different kind of memory? A deep sense of Someone Cared for Me.

Like a snake that knows the feeling of lying in the sun. Like an amoeba that moves away from being squashed to a place where nothing is squashing it. The part of Jason's brain that registered pain—which, on August 5, had failed Dr. Glass's pinch test—would also, I thought, recognize lack of pain, that is, comfort.

What did comfort mean to Jason?

Weight of a hand on his shoulder. Cadence and pitch of a beloved voice. Rhythm of a favorite song.

His memories, such as they were, would be discarded as soon as they were made, but maybe something would linger in his mind, some reptilian response that the world around him offered comfort, and like the snake returning to lie in the sun because yesterday that felt good, so Jason would come back to us—not in a few weeks or months but in the next millisecond.

The nurses taught us how to vacuum the phlegm that gathered, cobweb-like, around Jason's gums and in the back of his mouth and throat. Carefully we darted the suction stick into his tracheotomy. With swabs that resembled lollipops with square green foam tips, we caught the phlegm, twirling it around the foam like cotton candy. Sometimes we went too far with the stick, making him gag. Often, when we'd finished, after we'd extracted an astonishing amount of goo—the lubricant for his trachea and lungs, which, in a healthy active person, would be reabsorbed naturally—after we'd gone through an entire bag of swabs, Jason would sigh deeply, a sigh of contentment, a sigh that never could have gotten past the gobs of phlegm. Like this, we put him at ease. We helped him breathe.

He might not remember the banana or the basket of apples. He might not remember the hospital. But maybe he had a different kind of memory, a memory of that deep sigh, a memory lasting as long as a breath.

He was alive and therefore having some kind of experience. These days were something to him, though we could only guess at what that was, only try to interpret the smoke signals of his pulse and blinks, only try to make his reality one of comfort, free of pain.

The night Dr. Rooney said Jason would remember none of this, I dreamed I was holding Jason's hand as he lay in the hospital bed. He pulled me close and kissed me, putting his tongue in my mouth.

Tongue = language, I thought, still in the dream. How fierce is his desire to communicate. He is telling me that he is there.

Just a dream? Or was my mind translating a message, written in a language I didn't know I knew, stuffed in a bottle and tossed in the sea by Jason, who on some level remembered we were out there, believed we would receive it, trusted we would find him?

14

After my parents divorced but before they re-friended, we had some lousy holidays—arguments, walkouts, pinched cheer masking heartache, and one especially pathetic Christmas in which all attempts at ceremony collapsed and I found myself alone in a kitchen with a plate of blueberry pancakes, which I threw like Frisbees, one by one, out the twelfth-floor window. Since then I'd kept my expectations low.

Thanksgiving in the hospital was still and heavy yet accurate. The day didn't differ from the Wednesday before or the Friday after, except Jason didn't have any therapy sessions, so we stretched his arms and legs and feet and hands. Barbara Richardson and her husband invited us to their nearby apartment for turkey and pie. We went in shifts, so Jason would not be alone.

Like a tank, the holiday season rolled into New York. I dragged myself to the office party, squeezing into a pretty skirt, putting on makeup that only highlighted the pallor of my skin and the purple lines beneath my bloodshot eyes. By the time I reached the party, pouring rain had washed away the makeup as well as whatever resolve had convinced me to go in the first place, and I turned around and went home.

My birthday, in early December, fell on a Saturday, which in my mind meant I should have some kind of gathering. Muma offered her apartment, considerably larger than mine, and everyone was welcome—my friends, Jason and Monica's, Muma's, Rop's. We had cake and a song, but the occasion celebrated more than my turning thirty-two: the blessings that were Dr. Narayan and the many gifted and caring nurses and nurse's aides, the myriad sacrifices and efforts of the people at the party, the fact that Jason was alive and, at last, out of danger. With so many of his friends present, they almost formed his outline. He almost seemed to be there. But in the taxi heading back to Brooklyn, I cried for missing him. Funny, since I saw him now more than ever. But it wasn't his physical presence that I missed.

When Jason had arrived at Mount Sinai in September, Monica had met with the hospital's Medicaid liaison. Their health insurance, bought through Monica's job, had a per-person million-dollar cap. In other words, a million dollars was the maximum amount the insurance company would pay, over a lifetime, for each insured person. In August a million dollars had seemed like a distant, insurmountable number. How could he ever rack up a bill that high?

Easily. And the hospital knew it.

The liaison told Monica that because her salary was above a certain amount, she and Jason would not qualify for Medicaid. Her salary was not a fortune. Still, it was over a line.

Monica's stepmother, Jane, had worked for a lawyer in Boston who helped Medicaid applicants complete and file the necessary paperwork. From him Jane got the name of a Medicaid lawyer in New York. On December 7 Jane, Monica, and Monica's father, Lou, met with the lawyer. He echoed the Mount Sinai liaison: Medicaid would turn Jason down. But Monica could submit a Spousal Refusal Application, that is, she could refuse to make her income and assets available for Jason's care. On his own Jason would be eligible. This was not a slick trick to skirt Medicaid rules. The Mount Sinai liaison had made the same suggestion.

For Jason to benefit from society's safety net, Monica—employed, insured, pregnant with Jason's child, working full-time and coming to the hospital nightly—would sign a paper stating that financially she and Jason had split. On the one hand, as a procedure, the Spousal Refusal Application meant nothing. On the other hand, it epitomized Monica's Kafkaesque struggle to secure care for Jason. Already she spent hours on the phone with Eileen, the insurance rep, who questioned every treatment and refused many of them. With Jason, Monica had purchased insurance for an event such as this, only to discover that in an event such as this, the insurance company's goal was not Jason's recovery. Its goal was to pay as little money as possible. With no other option, Monica signed the application.

Using eight thousand dollars from the benefit concert, Monica hired the lawyer to make sure the Medicaid application was submitted properly. It wasn't. Two years later a bill for seventy thousand dollars would arrive, the first sign that the application had been bungled by both the lawyer and the hospital: Mount Sinai had reported an incorrect admission date, neither private insurance nor Medicaid would cover the ambulance on August 4, and the lawyer had delegated the job to a junior associate who left the firm, whereupon the application languished for months. But that mess was yet to come. Now the lawyer assured Mount Sinai that Jason would receive Medicaid, and at our weekly meeting Dr. Rooney effusively expressed his pleasure, assuring us that New York Medicaid was "great." We took his words to mean that Jason would be covered and Monica would no longer have to ask and argue and plead and be told no anyway.

One night the radio picked up WFUV from New Jersey—an old blues recording, a man singing and playing guitar.

"Jay," I said. "Is this Lead Belly?"

He made no motion.

"Jay," I said, "close your eyes if this is Robert Johnson."

Nothing.

"Jay, close your eyes if you know who is playing."

He closed his eyes.

Christmas was quiet. Jason slept all day. We passed presents over him. Through blinks Muma had figured out that Jason wanted her to buy Monica flowers. But Muma needn't have worried that Monica wouldn't receive a present from Jason.

"Just what I wanted!" Monica said, unwrapping a DVD box set of the *Lord of the Rings* trilogy, deftly stealing a page from his playbook. "Thanks, honey." She kissed him on the cheek.

I had wanted to find a present that Jason could use now. The options were limited. A book would be read to him. Clothes would be put on him. He had plenty of music. Rop was shaving Jason's face every few days, and hoping that Jason might participate, I gave him fancy shaving cream and aftershave. A few days later he dipped his crooked fingers into the cream and spread it on his face. The products were expensive, over my budget, but my feeling about money was like my feeling about food: why not indulge? And—it's for *Jason*. Look what he's going through. Doesn't he deserve high-end shaving products?

Monica unwrapped a wool coat, from her for him.

"For when you walk out of here," she said.

December 26. Minus five degrees outside. Ice on the sidewalk, salt in Lila's paws, the wind like a fist in one's face. Inside is a sauna, stuffy, thick with sleep. In the midst of it, Jason improves.

He raised a towel to wipe drool from his lips, rinsed his hands in a tub of warm water and dried them, nodded when asked if the song was "Double Trouble," signed his name on Rop's birthday card—his hand as tremulous as a seismograph, the tiny cramped script his, nevertheless.

"I love you," I said as I was leaving—I always said it when I left—and one night he blinked carefully, as if to say yes.

He wouldn't play a scale on the Casio keyboard, as Lou encouraged him to do, but instead tapped out a little melody using only two notes.

He pressed eject and removed the cassette tape, one of eight mix tapes sent by his friend Rod Alonzo, with all the songs in *MOJO* magazine's recent list of Fifty Best Guitar Solos, each introduced with commentary from Rod. He picked up the next tape, slid it into the slot, pressed play.

But these feats dotted days of sleep and lethargy, and victory's thrill was matched by worry. He moved as though through denser gravity. His hands shook. With his inklings of communication came increased expressions of pain. "Close your eyes if something hurts." He closed his eyes. I wanted him to respond, but knowing he was in pain made me sick. When he hadn't been able to convey anything, I had guessed at his inner state based on his pulse and breath and skin. Surely sometimes I had convinced myself he was all right.

December 28. The trach hole was plugged, and he made "ah" sounds and said hi.

With a cap now covering the trach at last Jason could work with the speech therapist. She asked us about his work as a musician. What did he play? What kind of music did he like?

Pulling up a chair in front of him, she said, "I want you to fill in the blank."

He showed no sign of acknowledgment.

In a plunking Long Island accent, with as much melody as if she were reporting the price of beans, she said, "The answer, my friend, is blowin' in the—"

She paused, waiting for Jason to say "wind."

He said nothing.

Later Muma, Rop, Monica, and I howled at the absurdity of her approach. But we were also at a loss. Rehab had fallen far short of our expectations, but what else could we do? We had no idea what other options were available or if other options even existed. We laughed, but we were also lost.

On January 7 Dr. Rooney said he was pleased with Jason's progress. He predicted a "full recovery." On January 13 Muma called me at work.

"Do you have a minute?" she said.

"Sure."

"Because it's bad news, and I don't want to tell you quickly."

"Go ahead."

"Rooney says he doesn't know how long Jason can stay at Sinai." The secretary to my right was on the phone with her divorce lawyer. "I want half," she was yelling. "You tell that SOB it's going to be thirty-nine hundred."

"I can't talk about this now," I said, and then, though I had listened dispassionately, somewhat not understanding, my inability to envision the future turning my mind blank, I burst into tears. I stood up. My calves hit the Aeron chair, sending it reeling.

"I love you," Muma said. She was crying.

I took a breath. "I love you too." I stumbled down the hall to the private bathroom, where I prayed on my knees, begging, demanding, "Don't abandon us!" I stood up, washed my face, and returned to my desk. My heart felt like it was going to blast my chest open.

"Are you all right?" asked the divorcing secretary. I didn't answer. It seemed like a water main had burst from one part of my life into another.

A few people at work knew about Jason. I wouldn't have given any details to the divorcée, but she sat next to me. "I couldn't do what you're doing," she'd said. She'd told me about bathing her mother, who was dying of cancer. Unable to face the withered shrunken body, she'd walked away, leaving her mother in the bathtub. "I couldn't do it," she'd said, and I had reminded her that she had been eighteen and alone.

"How's your brother?" another secretary asked, leaning over my desk. I hadn't mentioned anything to this woman, but word got around. "Is there a prognosis? Is there a date? When is the baby due? Well, I hope for a 100 percent recovery by the time that baby comes! Have a great night!"

No one could say the right thing, as far as I was concerned. I knew this and figured my best chance for the least disappointment was to say as little as possible. One colleague paused at my desk and said, in her Jamaican accent, "You look so sad lately."

Where to begin? "Hmm" was all I could reply.

According to Dr. Rooney, Medicaid would not keep Jason at Mount Sinai for longer than four weeks, after which he would be evaluated on a weekly basis. If he wasn't making enough progress, he would have to go.

Progress: the gun at our backs. If his progress stalled, if he *plateaued*, Medicaid would interpret it as indication that he had made all the recovery he could make and therefore no longer qualified to be in a rehab unit. But Medicaid payments lagged treatment by about three months. So if Medicaid decided that Jason should no longer be at Mount Sinai, it could stop payment, leaving Mount Sinai holding the bag. Sure, the hospital could try to collect payment from Jason and Monica, but if the money wasn't there, the money wasn't there. So Dr. Rooney was recommending that Jason move to a subacute rehab facility attached to a nursing home in Queens.

Four weeks?

Nursing home?

Queens?

We thought Jason was making progress. Did Medicaid understand the significance of his pressing PLAY on the boombox?

Of course hospitals must make money. Of course money is necessary. Still, it was—again, but as if for the first time—a harsh realization that Jason's care was driven not by what would help him but by cost.

Dr. Rooney's statement was shocking partly because he had given us no warning. One week earlier he'd said he was pleased with Jason's progress. Either he had openly lied or he had lied through omission. He didn't explain that *subacute* here was not an adjective but a classification, meaning the facility was not connected to a hospital. Nor did he clarify that the rehab program was separate from the nursing home. We heard *less intense*. We heard *nursing home*. We heard *the end*.

Later I learned that back in the Neuro-ICU one night, Monica was alone with Jason, who was then in very bad shape, and she started to cry uncontrollably. Two nurses held her for a long time. Eventually the head nurse arrived. "Why don't you come in tomorrow," she said, "and let's talk about the future." The next day Monica was told that the future for Jason would be a nursing home. Monica never relayed this conversation to Muma or Rop or me because she disagreed deeply with what the nurse had said and thought the rest of us didn't need to feel how she'd felt. But perhaps Dr. Rooney had seen this meeting noted somewhere and assumed we were discussing nursing homes—or whatever we were supposed to call them. *Skilled nursing facility, subacute rehabilitation program, nursing home*: for the uninitiated the jumbled language simply suggested *desertion*.

Dr. Rooney did not know or he chose to ignore that we believed Jason would make a full recovery. But we had said those words— with him, with everybody. *Full recovery*. He had said them too.

The doctor's suggestion was as abrupt and unacceptable as if he had told us to start calling Jason by a different name.

Hadn't Monica just moved from Brooklyn to Manhattan?

Didn't it already take Rop and me close to an hour to get to the hospital?

Queens?

He might as well have said Delaware. What was the place in Queens to us but far away?

Most surprising, most disappointing, most infuriating, was realizing that Dr. Rooney did not believe Jason would recover. He'd *said* he thought Jason would recover, but he hadn't believed it.

But who could confront him? Jason was in his care.

There was no reason for the doctor to have done anything differently. He was just part of the system, an unthinking, unimaginative, well-compensated cog.

The social worker handed us a trifold brochure for the nursing home, which listed Dr. Rooney as the facility's medical director.

So he was an unthinking, unimaginative, well-compensated *biased* cog.

Of course he would view the nursing home that employed him in a flattering light. There was no mention of other facilities that, if nothing else, might have been geographically superior.

What a racket. Not only had Jason's treatment been driven by money instead of recovery, but the money in question was not just insurance money, not just Medicaid money, not just money needed to run Mount Sinai. One set of hands in the pot belonged to Jason's doctor.

"We'll think about it," we told Dr. Rooney and the social worker.

Our answer didn't require any thinking. No way Jason was going to this place. But we would have to find the alternative on our own, and we would have to find it before Medicaid kicked him out.

15

Most of the notes in Jason's Mount Sinai patient record begin with the words "barrier to discharge." In other words, what's keeping him here? "Respiratory status," the notes say. Or sometimes "airway clearance." The clinicians hardly expected Jason to walk out. As soon as his respiratory status improved—that is, when the trach came out—he would go.

If we were in the dark about the clinicians' objectives, they were well aware of ours. "Pt's family continues to express their expectation that the pt will 'recover fully,'" writes the psychologist. She continued, "Sessions have involved pt's wife who appears better adjusted as evidenced by her less frequent tearfulness."

They wanted us to accept Jason's condition, to comply, to give up. I did not take for granted that Jason would recover completely, but I could not fathom denying him the opportunity.

After Dr. Rooney's about-face, we were done second-guessing our instincts.

In a window booth of a Madison Avenue diner we began to strategize. Perhaps it was strange that Monica, Muma, Rop, and I had not yet asked, What are we going to do? Since August 4, without discussion, we had known the answer—anything and everything. When he'd had meningitis and seizures, when he was in a coma, where else could he have been but in a Neuro-icu? Then care had meant survival. Now care had become a variable.

We knew nothing about rehabilitation hospitals. Our strategy was simply to find people who did.

U.S. News & World Report's annual ranking of top rehab hospitals listed a handful in the Northeast: Rusk (New York), Kessler (New Jersey), Gaylord (Connecticut), and Spaulding (Boston). As we were leaving Mount Sinai one night, Monica said Spaulding seemed to her the best choice. It was an excellent hospital, and her parents, divorced and both remarried, lived in the Boston area and could help with the baby, who was due in less than two months.

But how would Muma, Rop, and I see Jason? What about us?

A few days later the wife of a colleague, a neurosurgery resident at Yale–New Haven, spent about two hours on the phone with me. She suggested that we bargain with Mount Sinai: stop fighting for him to stay there longer in exchange for their pulling for Jason at the hospital of our choice. When I relayed the word *bargain* to the rest of the family, their ears pricked up. Even if we didn't really have negotiating power, we were emboldened by believing that the doctor, hospital, insurance, and Medicaid were no longer going to dictate Jason's future.

The phone call was the first time I had laid out Jason's course to a medical professional. As I explained the complications, his medications, our expectations, I realized that nothing was keeping me in New York. I could quit my secretary job and sublet my apartment. I had a little money saved, and at that point it seemed like enough to last for months. Once made, the decision felt preordained, a nondecision decision.

"I go where Jason goes," I said at our next family conference, and Monica said she was relieved to hear it.

Carnegie Mellon flew me to Pittsburgh to drop in on rehearsals of my play. The second plane was a puddle jumper. In the small outpost for connecting flights, I waited and waited. Five minutes before takeoff I approached the counter.

"What's happening with this flight?" I asked the woman there. "Are we going to board?"

"We've been calling your name for twenty minutes," she said. "You'd better hurry."

As if in a vacuum, I had heard nothing.

Insurance told Monica they absolutely would not pay for Spaulding.

"But this is his best chance at recovering," Monica argued.

"We won't authorize it," said Eileen.

A few conversations later Eileen said—in what could be the company motto—"I've recently learned that none of this matters." Jason had reached his lifetime cap.

New York Medicaid would never cover Spaulding, which was in Massachusetts.

At a loss, Monica called Spaulding's main number.

"How may I direct your call?" the receptionist asked.

"I don't know," Monica said. "I need some advice."

The receptionist, the best receptionist ever in the world, transferred the call to Marilyn Spivack, a pioneer in brain injury advocacy and support who had founded the Brain Injury Association of America. Monica introduced herself. She explained Jason's situation. "I'm going to help you," Marilyn said.

I took a train to Boston, the same train that Muma, Jason, and I had taken every Friday for so many years. When the train stopped in Old Saybrook, I thought of our family back then. Never in a million years could we have guessed where we would be now. Hadn't our story taken a strange sad twist. How I wanted a happy ending.

When the train arrived, near midnight, Jane was the only person in the cavernous station, and it occurred to me that my life of late had existed chiefly in desolate waiting rooms.

Spaulding, a smart *Y*-shaped brick building, sat on the banks of the Charles River, under the Zakim Bridge. The Brain Injury Unit was on the eighth floor, with two wings for patients, solariums at the ends of the halls, and a dining/activity room. On the other side of the elevators a third wing led to a library, a chapel, and a gym.

The guide talked about recreation therapy, a current events group, a sailing program, a mock car, a practice apartment, therapy dogs. The medical team, she said, would make a plan "to get the patient back to life before the accident." I stood quietly, trying to feel the vibe. Among the patients were men and women Jason's age. The floor buzzed with activity. "Positive and aggressive," I reported to Monica and my parents.

Marilyn Spivack made sure that in terms of logistics Spaulding would admit Jason. However, there remained the question of money. Who was going to foot the bill?

Everything felt crazy, and crazy felt normal. When a smoke alarm went off in an apartment on the second floor of my building and the super said he couldn't go in because the tenants were out of town, I picked up the phone to contact the building manager but instead called someone who would care. In three minutes firemen were clanking up the stairs with their tanks and axes. I opened my door to hear the super protesting—"If you had let me explain!"—and the chief's brassy rebuke—"This is the way we fight fires!"

"You can get to the backyard through my apartment," I told one of the men.

"We're already there," he replied.

Whack! Whack! Ax on a door. A man's voice: "Wrong apartment!" More whacks. Then at last silence.

Jane and Lou, who had been researching financing options, discovered that a person could declare himself a resident of Massachusetts after twenty-four hours in the state and, therefore, apply for Massachusetts Medicaid (aka Mass Health). But even if we could deliver Jason to Spaulding, there would be a transition period while his Medicaid application was being processed. Spaulding cost twenty-eight thousand dollars per month. If Mass Health came through, it would retroactively cover the transition. In the event that Jason was denied, Spaulding needed to know where its payment was coming from.

Even as we struggled to solve this riddle, Jason gained ground. He stood on his own using the parallel bars as everyone in the gym cheered. He played two notes on the piano gourd, back and forth. He put moisturizer on his lips. He indicated clearly that he wanted to hear *Peach Pony*, Rachel Loshak's new album. Mixing sessions had been scheduled for mid-August, and Rachel had agonized over finishing the project without Jason, but Monica had told her he would understand. No music drew his attention as did those songs. He played on all of them, and sometimes, drifting off while the CD continued, he twitched and jerked his arms as if playing guitar in his dreams.

On February 3 his trach came out.

A family friend, hearing about the twenty-eight thousand dollars conundrum, told Monica he'd been waiting for a moment to help. He would guarantee Spaulding one month's payment in case Mass Health did not take Jason.

Now we just needed a bed to open up.

"Jason's going to Spaulding," we said at our next weekly meeting with Dr. Rooney and the very tan social worker, who had recently returned from two weeks in Florida.

They looked at us like we were pitiful fools.

"I'll make some calls and see what I can do," said the social worker. Her voice made clear she was placating our delusions.

"You don't understand," we said. "He's in. He's going to Spaulding."

Their mouths fell open.

The moment was ours to savor, but it was also a perfect example of the medical system's sad division of haves and have-nots. We didn't have the money but we knew someone who did. If there hadn't been a family friend with thirty grand to spare, our options included the usual reasons for bankruptcy: going into debt, using up savings, cashing out retirement funds and life insurance policies. If none of those possibilities had existed, then Jason would have gone to some facility in Queens or elsewhere, or maybe he would have gone home and we would have made the best of it. Money gave us a viable choice. Judging from the shocked expressions of Dr. Rooney and the social worker, not many people without this kind of money managed to get ahold of this kind of choice.

Rachel Loshak had organized one more benefit concert in New York. Some of the nurses and therapists came to the sold-out show at Irving Plaza, which was headlined by Norah Jones and featured a roster of killer performers, all of whom knew Jason well. They played a lot of his music, and everyone joined in for "I Shall Not Be Moved," a gospel song that Jason loved. When Kenny White, alone at a grand piano, sang "Through Tomorrow"—one of my favorites, one of the first Jason had written—I gripped the balcony rail until my wrists ached. Not a weeper but a sobber, I cried in public only when surrounded by strangers, for I had seen friends disturbed by the intensity. No single tear down my cheek, no sniff-sniffing, no dabbing at my eyes. Rather, something closer to vomiting. I held in the turbulence.

Sometimes I glimpsed how I would crumble when this was behind us.

On a day when the phones and Internet went down and the office filled with the sound of conversation, I told my boss I was going to Boston. How long, I didn't know. He gave me a box of chocolates in advance of Valentine's Day and said he'd keep me on payroll if I thought I'd return. But I wasn't coming back.

Every day, every moment, I was waiting for the call.

On February 10 it came. Spaulding had a bed for Jason.

After leaving work for the last time, I stopped by Roosevelt Hospital to pick up scans of Jason's brain that had been sent to a neurosurgeon there months earlier, when we were exploring options for surgery on the AVM. We would need the scans to resume the search in Boston.

I was born at Roosevelt, a fact that, as I entered the lobby, gave me an acute perception of time. I could feel all the twists and turns of my childhood and adolescence and adult life, and it seemed equally odd and all right that they had been leading me here, to pick up scans of my brother's brain to take with me to Boston, where I was moving with him as he came back from the netherworld of this injury.

I walked from Roosevelt to Sinai by cutting northeast across Central Park. The sky was the royal blue of winter twilight. An installation by the artists Christo and Jeanne-Claude was being set up in the park. Over the paths stood sixteen-foot-tall rectangular gates, sometimes five or six in a row, from which would hang large brilliant orange flags. Through the bleak park I walked from one hospital to the next, following a winding route so I could pass under as many gates as possible. The installation would not open for another day or two. The gates were in place, but the orange flags were not yet unfurled—the final moment of something before it became something else.

16

Through the rear window of the ambulance I watched the New York skyline shrink, then disappear. I'd wanted to leave the city for years. But not like this.

Jason lay, strapped into a stretcher, wearing sweatpants and his red hooded sweatshirt, wrapped like a mummy in a blanket that insulated his emaciated body. He gave off a sweaty, yeasty smell.

"Blink if you're okay," I said a thousand times, and he blinked a thousand times.

My hand rested on his leg or arm or shoulder. If he forgot what was happening, at least he would feel human contact. Muma sat up front with the driver, who made the five-hour trip without stopping. Not designed for long-distance hauls, the ambulance engine strained as gusty winter winds blew us sideways. Somewhere ahead of us, Rop and Monica were with the cats in Muma's car. Somewhere behind us a moving van was taking to a storage unit in Newton everything from Jason and Monica's apartment except instruments, which Monica had distributed among friends for safekeeping.

The plan was for Muma, who had returned to teaching, to come to Boston on weekends; Rop would come up during the week. Monica would be at Spaulding as often as possible, but she was more and more limited by the last month of pregnancy, and soon she'd have her hands full with a newborn.

Earlier, while Muma, Jason, and I were waiting for the discharge papers, Dr. Narayan came to say good-bye. Muma thanked him profusely, but I turned mute, words and emotion colliding in my throat. If I tried to speak, surely I would start to cry—for gratitude, for fear—and if I started to cry, I would be unable to stop.

The night before, my neighbor Samara, who was taking care of Lila until I got settled, had given me a tarot reading.

"Tell me about the cute guy at the office," I'd said, afraid to mention Jason.

But the cards knew where my attention lay. "This is an affair of the heart," they said.

It was late Friday afternoon when Jason settled into his half of room 825, but a stream of people appeared at his door to introduce themselves and evaluate him. Nurses. Nurse's aides. Doctors. Residents. Therapists. They talked to him, adult to adult, respectfully, in a normal tone of voice. When the physical therapist asked Jason to raise his right arm as high as he could, he raised it higher than we'd seen since August.

"We're in Boston. We came to a different hospital," I told him around midnight, after peering over and finding him awake. The shadow of a nod crossed his face.

My makeshift bed—two armchairs pulled together—could not have been more uncomfortable, but I was too stirred up to sleep anyway. We had reached Spaulding. Jason was in the right place, and so was I. Now his recovery was my full-time concern. I wanted to be nowhere else, do nothing else. Because I loved him. Because I was angry at the cruel possibility that he might not know his child. Because somewhere in me was a confidence about how to get him back.

Many times in our childhood we'd had only each other for company. Summers, when we were too old for a babysitter, we had a nightly choice: stay home or go with Muma and Rop to the theater. Since we looked after each other, whatever our choice we made it together. We watched the show. Or played cards with actors in the green room. Or walked to the Sweet Suite for root beer floats. Or rolled in the dark down the steep grassy hill. Or we stayed home, where on Saturdays, while Muma and Rop ate with the company, we made our own dinner, heating something frozen in the toaster oven. We knew each routine, and because of this, in an unconscious, almost accidental way, we knew each other.

He had more nerve, or at least he learned before I did how to take action despite anxiety. At Goodspeed he was in *The Happy Time*, whereas I botched my audition for *Take Me Along*. During Hurricane Gloria he strolled across a low footbridge while I hesitated in the pouring rain, stuck wondering if this qualified as the kind of bridge we'd been instructed to avoid. Playing toy drum (him) and toy trumpet (me) in the Toy Symphony, part of a holiday concert, we approached a long rest according to our dispositions. I counted the measures; he listened for a certain cue.

After many summers at Bennett's, with its built-in gang of kids, we moved to a little yellow house on Lake Hayward, an abrupt clearing in a thick forest whose tangled bushes and crowded ferns seemed determined to grow back over the land cleared for driveways and lawns. The lake was twenty minutes from town, and our neighbors were old enough to have retired before Jason and I were born. We rode our bicycles around the lake, took the bike-a-boat through the lily pads, played Superman II (the board game) or Old Maid until, frustrated, I put a tiny tear in the old maid's card.

"This deck is ruined," he said.

"How did that happen?" I asked, with a straight face, fooling no one.

When we fought, he had the upper hand of age and strength and possessed a preternatural endurance that, through torture, he taught me. But I could scream and had a talent for playing the victim. We could go at each other and a moment later play Winter Olympics on our Odyssey video game console. The alternative was solitude.

94

After we moved from Lake Hayward into town, Jason and I found shortcuts to the main street via paths through the woods that, judging from the old map in the library, had been carved by mill workers whose ladies' boardinghouse had been where now stood our little apartment complex. When a man about two miles down the road opened a comic book store in his basement, we would walk there, browse for hours, and return, reading as we walked, silent except for the occasional cautionary "Car." Jason collected *X-Men, Spiderman, Fantastic Four;* I was *Archie* and *Mad Magazine.*

In our twenties we drifted apart.

"We didn't talk much when I was in California," I once said.

"You weren't always easy to reach," he said, correctly. Making up for that absence had partly motivated my decision to move to Boston. And I felt qualified. I was a certified EMT and had belonged to a volunteer squad in Brooklyn. I had an ear for medicine's lingo. One of my other jobs as I came up as a writer had been tutoring students, many of whom had learning disabilities, so I'd given much thought to how they processed information, to Howard Gardner's theory of multiple intelligences, to not presuming that my tutees would understand material the way I did. And being a writer, I'd spent a lot of time imagining life from the perspective of other people.

I was in Boston because I didn't want to miss the story.

One night we were hanging out in Rop's office, the show audible through the boxy brown speaker mounted on the wall.

"I'm going for a walk," Jason said.

"I'm staying here," I said.

I thought I knew where he would go. To DeLo's for potato chips, to the cemetery past the library, to the falling-down dock, to the tiny airport past the parking lot where years later Rop would teach me how to drive a stick, to the Victorian houses where actors stayed, to the scene shop and rehearsal hall at the far end of town.

Instead, he headed for the steel swing bridge that spanned the Connecticut River. He was halfway across when the bells rang and the red and white bars at either end descended. The bridge would turn.

"Come on up," called the man in the booth at the top of the bridge.

So Jason rode inside the booth as the bridge swung open. He saw the control panels. He watched from above as the tall boat sailed through.

When he told me this, I was jealous, filled with regret, left holding no more than the lesson: if you don't go on the walk, you'll never ride in the booth.

17

No more picking the banana from the basket of apples.

Also, no more phenobarbital.

Jason's new physiatrist, Dr. Heechin Chae, possessed a steady, accessible demeanor. He was a calm port after the storms of Mount Sinai. References to recent research often accompanied explanations of his decisions. With patience and few words he answered our many questions. Yet the doctor's observant, scientific manner did not mean he was afraid of risk. In fact, he took a distinctly unorthodox approach to Jason's treatment.

In Dr. Chae's opinion the seizures had been an isolated event. On scans taken after Jason's arrival at Spaulding, he saw evidence of previous bleeding but no fresh blood. Given the sedative effect of antiseizure medication and knowing Jason was surrounded by a watchful staff that would respond quickly if the seizures did return, Dr. Chae took Jason off phenobarbital. (Dr. Dear's replacement had reduced the dose significantly but not entirely.)

Increasing Jason's wakefulness was the central challenge. For although he had responded immediately to the direct respectful voices of Spaulding's therapists, still he was submerged, slow, often asleep; awake, he was like a tape playing at half-speed. His sluggishness was caused not just by phenobarbital but by the injury to his brain. Or, as Dr. Chae saw it, the *injuries*—

from the initial hemorrhage in the tectum of his midbrain, the blood like poison on the tissues it touched;

from the swelling that had followed the bleed and the swelling of the ventricles from the blocked aqueduct of Sylvius;

from the infection of the meninges;

from the seizures.

These events had damaged Jason's inner action. The mechanism that transmitted impulses into deeds was not functioning. Prolonged immobility had caused abnormally increased muscle tone—referred to simply as "tone"—which had tightened his joints: his mouth closed only with great effort, his wrists pulled forward, his elbows and knees rested bent, and his fingers folded over. Some fingers had been squeezed like this so long they'd lost the crease of skin between the lower two bones. But the tone would diminish if his brain could be roused. In other words, his barrier to movement—legs to walk, throat to speak—wasn't physical but cognitive.

Looking to stimulate Jason's brain, thereby giving the therapists a chance for engagement, Dr. Chae prescribed the dopamine-boosting medication amantadine. Originally an antiviral drug, amantadine had been found, following a flu outbreak, to reduce symptoms of Parkinson's disease, a discovery that led to its use in brain injury treatment. Dr. Chae hoped that more dopamine would mean more neurotransmitting. But rousing Jason wasn't a matter of simply goosing his brain.

Because depression can slow dopamine, an antidepressant was added.

Because Jason's pituitary gland had been damaged, leaving him with low testosterone, which contributed to fatigue and inhibited muscle buildup, testosterone was prescribed.

Also in the mix was Ritalin, which helped stir Jason's brain, though in Dr. Chae's opinion it was less effective than amantadine. Above a certain dose it made Jason's arms shake. Another drug stopped the tremors.

"Medication isn't magic," said Dr. Chae. It only gave Jason's brain a boost toward whatever potential for recovery existed. If the possibility wasn't there, it wasn't there.

Dr. Chae's use of medication was aggressive but justified, he felt, by the fact that Jason was six months post-injury. Phenobarbital notwithstanding, any spontaneous healing would have happened already. The time to wait and see had passed.

Besides, we had come to Spaulding because we believed that Spaulding's doctors would take calculated risks. If we had wanted to play it safe, Jason would be in the nursing facility in Queens.

"There is no standard of care in patients like Jason," Dr. Chae would later say. The norm was to sedate the injured brain as much as possible. As for how to raise the brain once the danger had passed—medicine was still figuring that out. Due to the risk-averse nature of doctors, many patients were left in a tranquilized state. "What I do is very maverick," Dr. Chae said, acknowledging other doctors' skepticism. "*Oh my gosh, you're risking someone having seizures.* My response is, don't you want to see if his brain will recover?"

He put us to work. Throughout the day we reported on Jason's condition, telling Dr. Chae when Jason's arms shook so he could fine-tune the Ritalin dose. Because we were there, he pushed Jason's medications.

At last there was a balance between what I was capable of doing and what I was being asked to do. Willing student and obsessive apprentice, I was at Spaulding morning to night, a sponge to the clinicians' every word. Once I was introduced by a doctor, jokingly, as an honorary resident, which sounded right.

The therapists set goals, broke them into smaller goals, further smashed them into manageable actions. One such goal was eating, which was addressed by speech-language pathology, the full name for what was often shortened to "speech therapy" and which covered not just speaking and eating but also language and cognition. For Jason to be able to eat, first he needed to swallow reliably. If he could swallow, he would not choke. To reach solid food, he would have to be able to handle liquids, and to reach liquids he would have to be able to swallow ice chips—safest because even if an ice chip lodged in the wrong place, it would melt. But, before the ice chip, the swallow. To wake up his mouth, Margaret, the speech-language pathologist, would rub his gums with a cold lemon-flavored swab. Again and again his Adam's apple would rise, with the back of his tongue still unable to make the final push.

Margaret often called me Kate, a name, she explained as she apologized, belonging to another sister who'd moved to Boston to help her brother at Spaulding. I didn't mind. In fact, I liked knowing that other sisters had sat in my chair as helpers, cheerleaders, witnesses. Being called Kate reminded me of the summer when I was fifteen. I'd played Katherine in *Taming of the Shrew* at Interlochen, and Kate had become my nickname. Margaret's mistake was like a messenger carrying memories of that fiery character and that summer when, as now, I'd felt daunted but sure I could take on the challenge before me.

Since Jason wasn't speaking, Margaret enlisted the Assistive Technology Department to outfit a board the size of a breakfast-in-bed tray with a buzzer and bell and switches and dials, which corresponded to various commands: *music on, music off, louder, softer, lights on, lights off.* Some of the sounds, such as the buzzer, were so sonically grating that Jason never would have used them, and by the time the board was constructed he was hushing out a whispery "hi," thus preempting the board's purpose. Nevertheless, Margaret's intention—to give Jason control of his environment— seemed as important as helping him eat and speak. *You're here. You decide. You have authority.* How easy and lazy it would be to press the opposite view—*you can't speak or move, so we will determine your world for you. You're incapacitated. You aren't really here.* It occurred to me that a person in Jason's situation was utterly malleable to whatever mind-set was offered.

His recovery, I was beginning to see, would both be conveyed to him and come from within him. In physical therapy he was put in a harness, like a rock climber's, attached overhead to a large walker—a Lite Gait—which suspended him upright. When Anne, the physical therapist, brought him to standing, he leaned on her shoulders, muscles shaking from the stretch and strain. A few sessions later she began advancing the Lite Gait down the hall outside the gym, while her assistant, Prima, sat on a low, wheeled stool, moving Jason's feet. The contracted muscles in his thighs and hips pulled his legs across each other like the first step in the Charleston, and Prima would pick up the foot and reposition it in the right spot. In this meticulous, laborious way they "walked" him, sending a message to his mind and body: *these movements, this coordination—remember?*

The PTs put casts on his legs, foot to thigh, first one, then the other, a novel kind of borrowing from another part of medicine, for his legs were not broken but they did need to be set and his bent knees held straight. After a week the cast was "bivalved": sawed in half vertically, cloth and tape over the rough edges, Velcro straps attached so it could be worn just at night, and I thought how pliable the human body was. He had fallen into a misshapen version of himself, but with a shrewd acceptance of the body's plasticity, Anne and Prima were guiding his legs back into their pre-injury form.

His hands were harder to mold. When casts proved too painful, the OT team made removable splints, and still the first splints—of dozens to come—could ask for only a very minor stretch. But the OTs were determined to bring his wrists back, millimeter by millimeter. A thousand actions would have been difficult or impossible with his hands left as they were: turning a doorknob, holding a fork or glass, punching numbers into a phone. The OTs—Mary, Nancy, Varsha—understood that Jason's hands were his livelihood, and at the same time they folded this information into the rest of the material they were gathering. Which hand was dominant? Did he use an electric razor or straightedge? To them ADLs—activities of daily living—were not a part of his treatment so much as clues to his identity. I started to understand that occupational therapy, which had so mystified me in New York, was the therapy perhaps most involved in the patient as an individual—not to say that the other therapists didn't treat Jason as an individual; they certainly did. But the fundaments of walking, speaking, or eating didn't *depend* on who the person was, whereas how a person put on a coat could be a telling detail of that person's demeanor. A person could go right arm first or left arm first, swinging the coat behind during arm insertion or letting the coat hang in front. Or get both arms in, low behind the back, and then shrug the coat on, or do the crossed-arms twist-over-the-head move from elementary school or raise the coat overhead and slip both arms in at once, like some men do with blazers. As in any book or movie or play, these gestures, these rhythms and routines, make a character. How does he brush his teeth? Does he put on pants before shirt, or vice versa? Sock-shoe, sock-shoe? Or sock-sock, shoe-shoe? Always double-knots the lace? To complete his morning routine—teeth, shave, hair—does he have a final action, one last muss, one last brush of his hand over his jaw?

Who was this patient? A mystery to be solved, a Gordian knot to be untied. Recovery was not about imposing a set of steps. To *recover* the person meant to help him be himself again, however that person now manifested or would manifest as recovery evolved. This approach required a lot of patience. The therapists at Spaulding had the patience of monks.

They were friendly, knowledgeable, experienced, tough. They pushed him. "Can you go farther? Can you try again?" They used us. As Jason and the PTs walked down the hall, Rop or Monica or Muma or I inched along with them, holding a towel to catch the drool that fell from Jason's mouth, pushing his glasses up his nose, softly cheering him on, fetching his wheelchair when he reached the finish line at the fire extinguisher so he could rest before returning. They made sure we knew the walk down the hall was for him like running a marathon. They taught us how and when to put on the splints and bivalved casts, how to transfer him between bed and wheelchair. They stressed that Jason needed a quiet environment in order to pay attention. Background noise, two people talking at once, too much information, could cause him to zone out. Keep him in touch with the outside world, they said, so we subscribed him to *Newsweek*, for its full-page pictures, and the large-print *New York Times*. Cards and letters from friends and relatives poured in with news of recordings, tours, babies, weddings, new jobs, new homes—life going on.

Spaulding was small, with three elevators and one staircase, and we met its community by passing people throughout the day, going up or downstairs, in line at the cafeteria, getting coffee at the Dunkin Donuts in the lobby. I would see Jason's therapists working with other patients in the hall outside the gym or in the solarium where the windows looked onto North Station, whose departure bells rang throughout the day, and the Suffolk County Jail, around which women stood in the evenings, sometimes with children, shouting conversations with men in the barred windows above.

As at St. Vincent's and Mount Sinai, it mattered to me to befriend not only the clinicians but also the receptionists and the security guards. At Spaulding, when the janitor and I greeted each other, he would remark on Jason's progress. So did Cecilia, who manned the patients' elevator, who knew without a word that I was going to the eighth floor.

There was the teenage boy shot in the head who wheezed a steady plaintive cry. There was the minimally responsive woman from whom paramedics had withheld oxygen because they thought she was faking her grand mal seizure. There was the man who grabbed at nurses and threw his feces against the netting that surrounded his bed and replied to anyone's hello with a snide, drawn-out "Fuck you."

Patients came and went, their families suddenly absent, but I suspected we would be fixtures. Jason's Mass Health application was approved, and every day was a flurry of phone calls to share a new milestone. He put a cone on top of a pole, wobbling but extending to his full height. He raised his trembling arms to embrace Monica. He reached out a finger—a motion so tiny it was almost indiscernible—and touched the soft fur of Jed Bear the dog.

My parents and I had moved to Boston with no idea where we would live, assuming that if we could get Jason to Spaulding, surely we could find housing—specifically, a two-bedroom, dog-friendly, not far from Spaulding, affordable, month-to-month lease or sublet. In the beginning Muma and Rop stayed with Monica's family and I was with friends in Medford, but we needed a place of our own. Our search became increasingly frantic—my philosophy about apartment hunting being that your place appears only after you've thrown yourself completely, madly, into the search; then again, our whole lives were now frantic and mad, and everything required throwing ourselves completely in—but we landed in an apartment owned by Monica's mother's cousins, currently empty because the hardwood floors had been redone. The short 150-year-old building on the corner of Harvard and Ellery, our temporary home, was solid and thick, made of brick and mahogany, with a bay window and a defunct but beautiful fireplace.

We covered every inch of the glossy floors with rugs from a discount store. From the storage unit, Monica lent us a couch, a bed, pots, plates, silverware, television. Cardboard boxes sat in the living room open just enough to find the kettle or frying pan. We took three chairs before realizing the dining table was at the back of the unit, beyond reach. Still we set the chairs in a circle, as if any day the table would arrive. Three chairs around an empty space struck me as the right set design for this play—a picture of the missing piece and the potential.

I lived suspended, with no more than clothes, some books, and my computer. My subletter in Brooklyn forwarded my mail whenever he felt moved to do so, which was infrequently. With Lila I wandered Robert Lowell's "humpback brick sidewalks of Harvard," marveling at the smell of smoke from a nearby hearth—fireplaces in the city being foreign to me—and my days had an airiness like the snow that fell and fell. I was unmoored, detached. Though I was in Cambridge for the arduous task of helping Jason, the move was also a relief, a break from the grind of New York. Daily plans simplified. Rather than go to a job and then go to the hospital, my job was to go to the hospital. The hours I'd spent on the subway disappeared into the past as I drove Muma's car to and from Spaulding, with Lila curled up in a pile of sleeping bags in the back. I was doing exactly what I wanted to be doing, so despite the fact that what I was doing was hard and heavy and scary, my all-in participation yielded a satisfaction so deep it could almost have been called happiness.

I knew Boston and Cambridge barely from a handful of trips: in 1982 Rop had conducted *Little Johnny Jones* in out-of-town tryouts before Broadway, where it closed after one performance; in 1988 Muma and I had helped Jason move into his grungy freshman dorm at the Berklee College of Music; and in 2001 Jason and Monica's wedding had taken place somewhere in Cambridge. None of those memories could tell me where to walk Lila, buy groceries, get coffee, get gas, park the car. With the area all but new to me, ordinary tasks became adventures. I kept a map in my pocket and learned the North End, the different bridges that crossed the Charles, landmarks, thoroughfares, shortcuts. Roads named on paper were often in reality a number—Monsignor O'Brien Highway or Route 28?—and, as if by tradition, signs appeared ten feet after they would have been useful. But commenting on this and the locals' obnoxious driving and nerdy obsession for shorter routes—*I took Cambridge instead of Mass. Ave. and brought the drive down by forty-one seconds*—was part of the move we had made. Jason's treatment had changed radically, and we, too, had leaped from our New York routine, and every moment that the decision proved not a mistake felt like glory, and some moments were sublime.

In the hall outside the gym Jason, Anne, and Prima advanced toward me in the Lite Gait. Dr. Chae approached and stood behind me, watching.

Then he said under his breath, almost to himself, "He's breaking through."

18

In Spaulding's eighth-floor chapel, which was actually just half a conference room cut by a folding wall, I found the *Dhammapada*, a book of Buddhist scriptures, whose pages I flipped to read verses at random.

> If, with perception polluted, one speaks or acts
> Thence suffering follows
> As a wheel the draught ox's foot.

I copied these words onto a yellow Post-It fished out of my wallet, the only paper on hand, which Dr. Narayan had given to me on one of our last days at Mount Sinai. At the top of the slip, like an incongruous title for the ancient text, was Jason's shunt type: RADIONICS LOW PRESSURE VALVE.

The passage was an important reminder, for despite my enthusiasm for Spaulding and my delight at being liberated from dark hard New York, rampant criticism filled my mind. My confidence in helping Jason sometimes spilled over into unfair, unfounded judgment. When someone said or did something that didn't fit with my vision for his recovery, I scoffed.

These thoughts were, as the first line said, *polluted*. After all, I was no expert. The passage was both statement and caution. If you speak or act based on these thoughts, you may hurt someone's feelings, bring discord into the group, drive people away, or be filled with regret. One way or another, suffering will come.

I stifled my disapproval. If the pollution could not yet be cleared, perhaps it could be contained. I was constantly holding back, monitoring, keeping myself in check.

If one, though reciting little of texts,
Lives a life in accord with dharma,
Having discarded passion, ill will, and unawareness,
Knowing full well the mind well freed,
He, not grasping here, neither hereafter,
Is a partaker of the religious quest.

These words—same chapter, later verse—which I squeezed onto the back of the Post-It, the last lines crawling up one side, were like guidance for an oath I'd taken without knowing it.

Religious quest nailed how I felt about the move to Boston, the long hours at Spaulding, everything we'd done since August 4. Jason's recovery was our holy grail, and though we didn't know how to find it, we knew we would spend everything trying. The arduous, tortuous undertaking was leading us beyond the ordinary, beyond splints and medications, and my devotion was as earnest and immersive as a novitiate's.

And while I could read books about the brain and articles on rehabilitation, the real work lay in watching the therapists, the nurses, and Jason and in doing what was called for—holding a towel, bringing the wheelchair, or just showing up, the latter a particular challenge, considering the long stretches of boredom, the ugly sight of suffering, the awful reason for being there in the first place. The desire to escape somehow, at least through the mind, could be overwhelming.

But to live *in accord with dharma* was to face the phenomenon— the truth and the mystery—of Jason's injury. Not wishing it hadn't happened. Saying only that today he put a cone on the pole. Today he shook.

Today. How difficult, but how necessary, to focus on Jason's state today while not taking today as a blueprint for his future. I wanted his recovery. I could not control his fate.

But I could recognize this wanting and try to let go, try to accept Jason's path and my role *in* it, not as commander *of* it; accept that Jason's well-being did not depend upon his deserving more or less than other patients or my repulsion at the thought of him being this limited forever.

If I was not quite the partaker of the religious quest described in the *Dhammapada*, I could at least turn in its direction. Sometimes I found myself reoriented by circumstances, as by the class Spaulding offered every Wednesday to help families better understand how the brain worked.

Our class was led by Dr. Chae. For reasons of confidentiality he couldn't use patients' names, but his description of Patient A gave me a sinking feeling, not because I recognized Jason—clearly he was Patient A—but because, hearing Jason's deficits stated in the third person, I realized that his condition was far more severe than I had allowed. My flu shot a few months earlier had required a doctor's note because of a vaccine shortage. "Jason Crigler sustained a life-threatening hemorrhage in his brain," began Dr. Narayan's letter, words that made my stomach flip. Life-threatening? Of course, but to read it terrified me. I could grasp reality, but to function I had to deny it. Half a year after Jason's injury, still I knew and didn't know.

February 28. Maybe I have been kidding myself. It is such a serious injury. It's right in the middle of everything. Which just makes me wonder, how far back can he come? Two times in two days I have heard the advice: don't get caught up in the future—you cannot predict it.

During an examination of Jason's eyes, Spaulding's ophthalmologist referred to Jason's "stroke."

"He didn't have a stroke," I said. "He had a brain hemorrhage."

"A hemorrhage is a kind of stroke," said the occupational therapist who was in the room with us.

I could count on one hand the number of days since August 4 that I hadn't been with Jason. But I had not heard anyone use the word *stroke*.

I had heard *brain injury*, a clunky term, far less lyrical than *neuro* or *head*.

In fact, *stroke* refers to any loss of blood to brain cells, whether because it's leaking out of an artery or vein or is blocked by a clot or for some other reason.

If my not-knowing sometimes led to awkward moments, in other ways it contributed to a belief in infinite possibilities.

"The brain is the final frontier of medicine," said Dr. Chae at our Wednesday class. We have a good understanding of the other organs, but much about the brain remains undiscovered.

We don't know what it's like to be in that twilight state.

Barbara Richardson's words from months ago remained with me. I still felt comforted by a doctor saying *we don't know.* Because if medicine and science had yet to figure out how the brain worked and how it healed, then no one could tell me with certainty that Jason would not recover.

He was presented at rounds, in which a prominent neurologist from a nearby hospital would hear the case, then ask questions and share his thoughts with the audience. About a hundred clinicians attended.

Jason's therapists spoke. The neurologist reviewed some of the brain scans. Then Jason was brought in. The neurologist asked him to speak, stick out his tongue, lift his leg. Jason responded but not fully. He whispered "hi," but more like "huh," as if he were fogging a mirror.

Seated in the middle of a row, I fought the urge to rush to his side. He'd perform better if someone could remind him why he was in front of all these people. But I felt small and shy and made of lead. Soon he was taken out.

Maybe I didn't want the information sugarcoated.

"Considering the number of factors involved, there are questions that will probably never have an answer," the neurologist said. "The bleed. The swelling of the ventricles. The infection."

He continued: "Arousal and motivation mechanisms are in the brain stem"—where Jason's AVM was located—"and in studies wherein this area was shut off in rats, the rats starved to death because they had no motivation to eat."

He told the story of a man in the 1880s who had been hit in the head, unable to function or speak, whose son asked, "Where are the tools?" The man managed to say, "Master's."

"You have to imagine the terrific significance for the family's well-being of locating the tools," the neurologist said.

So Jason's rehabilitation would be more than stretches and muscle building, more than casts and exercises. It would involve motivation. Not just *feeling* motivated but reaching the *seat* of motivation, the place where something I understood as abstract—part cerebral, part emotional—was a tangible group of cells.

I could hardly think of anyone more motivated than Jason.

If his motivation had been knocked out, then we would provide surrogate motivation until his returned. We would want for him, get for him. His motivation was palpable—when we said, "Close your eyes if you want to listen to another chapter of Dylan's memoir," he closed his eyes; he whispered "Yeah" when Anne asked if he could do another lap down the hall—but he was unable to call upon this force at will. Fatigue descended upon him like a blanket, and then his motivation flickered, tamped down, almost extinguished.

"After an injury the brain has to form new pathways," the neurologist said. "When an old pathway is wrecked—from the initial bleed, say—the brain reroutes, the same way that when a highway is under construction, drivers take local roads. Over time the temporary path becomes the new highway."

A few days prior, Rop and Muma had spent a good ten minutes greeting Jason over and over.

"Hi," one of them would say.

"Hi," Jason would reply.

"Right," Margaret had said when she'd heard about it. "He has rediscovered the neural pathway for saying hi, coordinating respiration and forming the word with his mouth."

"I can't tell which way this will go," the neurologist said. Seven months had passed since the injury. The standard window of opportunity was six months. After that a patient was expected to plateau. But Jason had had so many complications after the bleed that it was hard to pinpoint the start date.

The window of opportunity slammed shut on my fingers.

The plateau, endless expanse, was Siberia.

I can't tell, the neurologist had said.

We don't know, Barbara Richardson had said.

The window and the plateau were meant to signify how much progress Jason would make—which, the doctors admitted, they really couldn't predict.

Progress. That other tired term.

Who had coined these phrases—doctors or insurance companies? Observation or self-fulfilling prophecy? Surely whoever settled on *plateau* and *window of opportunity* was not someone for whom practice was a daily part of life—not a musician or writer or meditator—the key being to show up because otherwise you're done. Progress, sure. But first, intention.

Standing in the hall after rounds, I watched the crowd disperse. What if the plateau *was* progress? What if a patient was always making progress, even tiny increments, for the rest of his life? Then the plateau would be not a stopping point but infinite improvement.

Seeing the plateau as progress changed the goal from a finish line to a way of thinking. Jason was there but submerged. For insurance companies and many doctors, this was enough. They didn't need or want to know more. But we sought to understand and resolve a deeper question. Regardless of the parameters of the medical establishment, how could he recover? Forgetting cost and expectations, forgetting even the history of brain injury medicine—how could he get back?

He would recover by never ceasing to recover.

As long as there was progress—even the smallest amount at the slowest pace—his rehabilitation continued.

The amount and the speed of his improvement mattered less than the existence of *any* amount, at *any* speed.

This idea seemed the rehabilitative iteration of Newton's first law of motion: a body in motion stays in motion.

It was a version of Heraclitus's observation that the only thing constant is change.

If progress was Jason's plateau, he would always be reclaiming a little more of his life. He would be recovered not when he could perform certain activities, not when the "barrier to discharge" had been cleared, but when he himself could keep this motion in motion, cause his own change, throw open—throw away—the window and set out across the plateau of more progress and more progress and more.

19

"The brain is lazy," said Dr. Chae at our last Wednesday class. "It doesn't want to recover."

In a cut, blood coagulated, a scab formed, skin rebuilt itself. The fabric of bone could sew back together after a break. Not so for the brain, apparently. I remembered walking into Jason's room at Mount Sinai and seeing him in his wheelchair, inert and mute, and while several factors were at play—medications chief among them—it seemed reasonable to believe that his brain, left to its own devices, would not recover like skin or bone.

If his brain was lazy, then we would be industrious on its behalf.

Full-court press echoed in my mind as we read to him, played books on tape, played music, stretched him, repeated PT and OT exercises, clocked his time in casts and splints, held up magazines, read cards and letters from friends. Once a week a massage therapist worked on him, giving his body a different kind of treatment, offering him a break and reward.

To Monica's parents it looked like Rop, Muma, and I were smothering Jason. The difference of opinion edged into conversations, finally making its way to the rehab psychologist, Dr. Christopher Carter, who invited the families to meet with him.

Your circumstances are strange and difficult, said Dr. Carter, with everyone gathered in the solarium. Not only Jason's injury but the move from New York. Financial strains. Baby due in days. You're in-laws who have known each other to a limited extent. Among you are divorces and remarriages. And now you're thrown together in this collective effort.

He asked us each to identify what we could and could not do in this situation.

To my surprise, some people said they hated hospitals and preferred to avoid Spaulding. Some saw themselves helping Monica with the baby. Some would track hospital bills and communicate with lawyers and insurance. Some would help Jason.

Defining our roles was like letting the air out of an overstretched balloon. Fearful, new to this, with scant time or energy to plan how best to work together—or even to recognize that we *were* working together—we'd become muddled. Jason and Monica's marriage may have introduced us, but fate had made us something other than in-laws. Understanding our new roles meant taking on yet another task—but that was easier than the cloudy vagueness under which we'd been operating. Distinct families when we'd entered the meeting with Dr. Carter, we emerged more like a clan.

On the subject of smothering-versus-stimulation, Dr. Carter agreed that at this point Jason needed intervention. An aggressive approach was further confirmed at a meeting on March 1 with Jason's entire family and medical team. All therapists reported progress. He was reaching for the bed rail. He was sequencing. He was problem solving. He was turning his head in the direction he wanted to walk. He had graduated from the Lite Gait to an Atlas Walker: no more harness holding him up. Where he was stuck—still not swallowing, for example—the therapists outlined their next tactic. We asked what could be done about his eyes, what was happening with his hands, about surgery on the AVM.

He would not walk out of Spaulding the man he'd been before the injury, but the therapists offered a picture of Jason leaving needing minimal assistance, with the long view of achieving independence or something close. No one made any promises. Their language straddled hope and caution.

Then Dr. Chae said he was recommending that before going home Jason transfer to a skilled nursing facility (SNF: "sniff").

How long could he stay at Spaulding? we asked.

Six to eight weeks, probably.

How long would he be at the SNF?

About four months.

I had signed my agreement to go where this took me. One more hospital was one more obstacle on the course. And yet Dr. Chae's recommendation revealed Spaulding's prediction for a limited recovery. These clinicians, whose opinions I trusted implicitly, who moments earlier had attested to Jason's progress, did not believe he would come all the way back. I felt homesick, wishing desperately to return to the time before all this happened. Not because of the step-down facility, not because the meeting had changed my convictions, but because again we were alone. We would take from Spaulding everything we could get, and it would be a lot, and then we would set out again.

At least in the conversation were the words I'd been waiting to hear since the beginning: *going home.*

20

"Ben, Adam, Alex," Muma said.

"Mark," I said. "Brian, Paul."

While Jason lay in bed, silent but awake, we were trying to list all his elementary and high school classmates. Some boys we'd known for years, through Thanksgiving dinners, joint birthday parties, sleepovers, their parents friends with Muma and Rop, their sisters my schoolmates.

We switched to teachers. Miss Yellin in first grade. Mr. Thurman for music. What about the time a boy removed the ringer from the bell used by a teacher to call the class to order? Or the time a boy stuck a pair of tweezers in a socket, setting off a minor explosion?

"Who was your senior advisor?" Muma asked. "An Italian name." She went through the alphabet, asking Jason to close his eyes when she reached the first letter of the advisor's name.

M.

"Maglione," Muma said, mispronouncing what should have been a silent *g*.

In a soft voice Jason corrected her. "Maglione."

And with that his voice was back.

Just in time. A few days later he sat in his wheelchair in the hall outside the gym, about to stand, when the call came on my cell phone.

"Hello?" I heard Monica say. I passed the phone to Jason, who took it with a quick sure hand.

"Hello?" he said loudly.

"Jay, I'm here with our daughter," Monica said.

"Are you okay?" he said. "What's she doing?" Then, "I love you."

When he hung up the phone, a small crowd surrounded him. Knowing from the ultrasound that the baby was a girl, Monica had been meeting with Jason in private, reading lists of names, asking him to blink when he liked one.

"What's her name?" Muma and I cried out.

"Ellie," he said.

A line of well-wishers formed to shake his hand, and he accepted each congratulations with a clear "Thank you."

Anne helped him to his feet. "The victory lap," she said. Together they walked down the hall and back, at a faster clip than ever, and he needed less assistance keeping his legs from crossing over each other. "You should have a baby every day," she said when they returned.

Spaulding offered its chair car, a van outfitted to accommodate wheelchairs, so Jason could visit Monica and Ellie at Brigham and Women's. Rop and I went with him. It was Jason's third time outside since August.

Monica had been given a palatial room. Every surface held a vase of flowers. Jason was quiet, perhaps overwhelmed by the number of people in the room and the bustle and excitement. Or did he not understand where we were and why?

Two weeks later Dr. Carter would test Jason's memory by asking, "What major event recently happened in your life?" and Jason would say, "I don't know," but would recognize the answer when offered as multiple choice. In Monica's hospital room he was as present as he could be.

Into our bitter circumstance came an innocent baby, not just happy but seeming to be made of joy, as if some magical alchemy had turned Monica's tears into glee. To look at Ellie was to know that the indifference of life can also put beauty into a monstrous situation.

A colossal relief—Ellie born, and both she and Monica were healthy. Still, as Rop and I wheeled Jason back to the chair car, I felt like we were moving not through carpeted sunlit halls but across a frozen lake whose icy surface was ready to crack.

March 8. I am afraid the AVM will rebleed and Jason will die. I am afraid we will be thrown from the cliff of happiness to the rocks of grief.

He drank orange juice, in six months the first flavor other than lemon swabs to cross his lips.

"How does it feel?" I asked.

"Like seeing an old friend."

His voice was a quiet monotone. The muscles around his ribs and diaphragm had atrophied. He couldn't draw a deep breath. His tongue was slow. The tightened muscles in his face restricted his jaw and lips. But he was beginning to talk in full sentences, asking real questions, engaging in conversations.

"It's good to see you," he said when Margaret entered his room.

"That's not the usual response I get from people," she said, bemused.

What a tremendous achievement, to speak! And how distressing to discover what lay beneath. He could forget an event a minute after it happened. He was frequently down. While he had been mute, we could assume he wanted our help, but what if he didn't? What if his short-term memory never recovered? What if there was no relief for his depression?

He never sounded more like his old self than when friends visited. Some came from New York, making the round trip in one day. Some were passing through town for gigs. Especially when the subject was music—albums, gear, news from the downtown scene—Jason's voice seemed fueled by an old familiar energy.

Kenny White stopped by, and, looking for a place to hang out, they wound up in the patient dining room, which doubled as an activity room and so had board games, a TV, and, against a wall, a piano. Kenny began to play "Through Tomorrow," Jason's song, which Kenny had performed at the Irving Plaza benefit concert. He started but blanked on the lyrics. In a faint, fragile voice, Jason sang the rest.

Hearing this, we exploded with happiness. *Jason! Singing!* Whatever else we would find in his mind—confusion, sorrow, black holes—music was there too, *his* music, and this seemed the surest sign that the Jason we knew was alive, if not entirely intact.

21

If Jason was more like himself when he was around his friends, I felt increasingly alien among mine. When I moved to Cambridge, I knew three people in the area. At a birthday party for one of them, everyone seemed fluent in a language I didn't know. Witty, buoyant, loud, they summarized their lives in one neat sentence about work, graduate school, marriage, children. My voice sounded strange, as if I were hearing myself talk for the first time in months. I had no neat answers for their questions about Jason. I was doing something else, hard to explain, no predictable date of completion, and the solitude of my choice kept me apart.

March 15. I feel like a skiff in a squall. Where am I? Afloat, yes. Going somewhere, yes, somewhere unknowable.

Mornings Lila and I walked across Harvard Yard and the Cambridge Common to circle around the wide yellow Longfellow House, George Washington's headquarters at the start of the Revolutionary War. Under a big tree we would stop, she chewing on a stick while I wondered what had gone through Washington's mind when he lived here. What had he seen? How much was the same? Very little, I figured. Still, I would try to find one thing that the both of us might have looked at. The river. A corner of the house. The curve of Brattle Street.

One day the dog and I followed a different route home and emerged at the Episcopal Divinity School, whose Gothic archways and stained glass, from a distance, were vaguely familiar. The memory clicked into place. Jason and Monica's wedding was held in this chapel. I peered through the windows of the cafeteria next door, where they'd held the reception. In the empty room I could see the crowd of revelers dancing in a circle to "We've Only Just Begun." The band, the strings of light, the long tables with white cloths and Mason jars of flowers were as real to me as the glass against which I leaned. As if the past were present, I saw the scene. Was I simply experiencing the passage of time? Was the vision an offshoot of nostalgia, an emotional manifestation of you-never-know-where-you'll-end-up? Four years after your beautiful wedding you may be in a hospital relearning to walk, you may be giving birth to your child in your husband's absence. The feeling was the fulcrum between the not-knowing of the past and the knowing of the present. Standing under the tree next to Washington's house I would think of the general who could not have known the course of the Revolution.

After my parents left Goodspeed, when I was home from college, I would drive Muma's car to East Haddam. With a skeleton key that had never been returned, I would wander through the theater that felt so much like an old friend. *Still here.* My years at Goodspeed had ended so abruptly that sometimes they seemed not to have taken place at all. Sparkly cement back stairs, low knobs on the dressing room doors, lump on the pole in the green room, blue velvet seats: to see and feel these parts gave me some assurance, a bridge from present to past.

In New York, not long before the move to Boston, I'd gone to see a movie. When it was over, I watched the audience step up the aisle. One woman looked familiar, then a man, and I wondered how many times I'd seen a movie in the same theater with someone I'd known years ago but we'd missed each other—in the dark, absorbed in our own thoughts, not searching for old acquaintances.

Then again, on the subway platform that night, someone with an almost familiar face. I was surrounded by ghosts.

Perhaps this heightened sense of time and place helped me imagine Jason's current there-and-not-there-ness. I was comfortable meeting him on that frequency. But to dwell too long in that zone meant I was disengaging from the material world.

March 10. Are we here? Part of me is not. I would like all parts present.

Muma had enough mileage points on United to fly me to Pittsburgh to see my play at Carnegie Mellon. I left at dawn, caught the matinee, flew back that night. The play had been workshopped at a number of theaters, but this was its first full production. After the show, as I thanked the cast and crew, I was my old self—a writer putting work out into the world.

The director and I cruised around Pittsburgh until my return flight. As we rode up the Duquesne Incline, I found myself wondering, if Jason could not realize his dreams—if he would not play the guitar again, if he had to live in some kind of facility—how would I justify pursuing my own?

But why shouldn't I? And who was to say whether or to what degree Jason would succeed?

Home late, as I pulled back the blanket to slip into bed, it seemed impossible that since morning I had gone to Pittsburgh and seen a production of a play I wrote. It was easier to think the day had been a dream.

22

Nestled in a woods behind a loosely developed suburbia sat a squat brick building, inside which were fake flowers and pictures of flowers and mauve-and-tan wallpaper with a flower motif. In the lobby I watched a young woman in terry cloth sweatpants with a logo across the seat present a young man in a wheelchair with a bouquet of balloons.

Jason had been at Spaulding eight weeks. It was time to decide on a discharge plan. We'd driven an hour outside Boston to look at a highly regarded skilled nursing facility.

In a library that doubled as a conference room, Monica, Rop, Lou, Jane, and I met with a man and woman who were kind, professional, and overweight. The man, an administrator, was young, with a soul patch that struck me as deliberately scraggy. Why shouldn't he have a scraggy soul patch if he could do his job?

Soft peanut butter cookies and soda were offered on a tray, and coffee, which we declined, but the soul patch poured himself a cup and I had the sense that he didn't know he was going to be in this meeting until he'd arrived at work this morning.

Again I scolded myself. Surely these were professional, responsible people.

We asked questions about insurance, quality assurance, activities, therapies, visitors' hours. The answers were straightforward.

"We've seen patients leave in as little as four months," the woman said. Activities included "the Bingo" and trips to Walmart. There were no obstacles to Jason's coming here. "That's the one good thing I can say about this company," she said, explaining that the SNF accepted patients with any kind of insurance. The *one* good thing she could say? I knew what she'd meant. Still, I winced.

Our questions exhausted, we took a tour. Waiting for the group to assemble, I stood at the entrance to a large room full of patients who had come for Barn Babies, a monthly event. The visiting animals included ducks and dogs, but I was more interested in the facility's population, conveniently gathered.

There were people with Down syndrome, people who appeared minimally responsive, people with portions of their brain missing: gaps in the skull shape. Some slept. Some sat with their mouths open, drool falling out.

I imagined Jason taking a place among them. Here perhaps he would decline to be someone staring at a wall. He had, after all and not long ago, been someone seemingly "lost in space." But he was not now that man.

I had already decided that I would do anything to prevent Jason from coming here, but still I wanted to assess the place fairly. Could I look at this facility as *an* option, not *the* option? Could I take Dr. Chae's recommendation seriously and develop a measured response?

We saw dank rooms with cinderblock walls. We were taken through doors locked and armed for alarm.

"Don't worry. No one's going to reach out and grab you," said the soul patch as we passed through the wing for ambulatory patients. In the gym, where two men painted a window's trim, he explained, "Some patients need something to do." He brought us to a room where, after completing various tasks and activities, patients could redeem points for a reward. In the near-empty room I saw Barbie dolls, jigsaw puzzles, shaving cream.

April 7. What, and to what extent, are the patients recovering? They recover toward what the people around them think is enough. And what is enough? We are working to help Jason recover in a way that maintains his life's inherent loveliness. I think that has driven our philosophy of recovery: that Jason not just recover his health but that life be beautiful for him—not in a passive way but that the beauty of life that he already found for himself and contributed to in many ways—that *that* should guide the recovery. It's not just about phenobarbital levels.

We told Dr. Chae that Jason would come home. To our surprise, the decision bought Jason a few more weeks at Spaulding. Skilled nursing facilities like to have a tangible goal when the patient arrives, so acute rehab hospitals discharge patients a little "ahead of time." (Unsurprisingly, this is an insurance-driven setup.) The therapists shifted their objectives to helping Jason transition home.

His checkout date was mid-July.

The decision set more wheels turning. What home was he going to? Would we have help? What kind of equipment would we need?

"Are you sure you know what you're getting into?" Dr. Carter asked.

As was our way by then, we said yes and charged forward. We had no idea what we were getting into—we couldn't have—but we knew for us no other option existed.

One Saturday afternoon in early April we signed Jason out and went to Lou and Jane's house in Cambridge for lunch. He was, at last, eating. Wanting him to remember rich and fabulous food, I had been buying him mango lassis from India Palace and chocolate milkshakes from Burdick's. He deserved more than standard hospital fare, and I wanted to protect his mind from forgetting the pleasures and possibilities of food—and life—beyond room 825.

We had been bringing the world into his room. Now he was stepping out into the world.

With the weather warmer, every day we took Jason to Spaulding's small riverside park. He went with us to meetings with potential neurosurgeons. Finally, he was stable enough to undergo surgery on the AVM. Because it was located so deep inside his brain, traditional surgery—cutting through tissue—would do more harm than good. A better course was proton beam radiation, in which protons, fired at the AVM, would pass innocuously through brain matter to reach and obliterate their target. Jason didn't say much in the meetings, but we made sure he was there. We watched how the neurosurgeons treated him. Did they talk to him or to us about him? The neurosurgeon we ultimately chose—Dr. Paul Chapman at Massachusetts General Hospital, working in collaboration with Dr. Christopher Ogilvy—began the meeting by saying to Jason, "I want to apologize in advance, because I am going to talk about you in the third person even though you are right here."

But on this sunny Saturday afternoon in early April we were going with Jason not to another hospital, not to an appointment with a neurosurgeon, but to a house near Central Square. Lou, Jane, Jason, Monica, Ellie, Muma, and I sat outside eating sandwiches from Carberry's. The normalcy of it was stunning.

"What a great day!" Muma said when we were back in Jason's room at Spaulding.

"What did you guys do?" he said.

Any memory of the trip, the sunshine, the sandwich—already gone.

Another Saturday I sat by his bed flipping through the *Phoenix* when my eye fell on a listing. Bluegrass legend Ralph Stanley and his Clinch Mountain Boys were playing the Sanders Theatre that night. Muma called Monica. Yes, she could meet us there.

"He must be back by midnight," the nurse said. He was a latter

-day Cinderella. If the paperwork looked like he'd been out overnight—if, say, he returned at 12:01 a.m., technically the next day—Mass Health might ask questions like, Why does he need to be at Spaulding if he can be out overnight?

Bringing Jason to the Sanders Theatre was like a pilgrimage to healing waters. Made of old wood and stained-glass windows, the house boasted acoustics best described as divine. To hear Ralph Stanley live anywhere would be phenomenal; to hear him here was exceptional, a fact everyone in the audience knew, giving the energy around us an electric charge.

After each song Jason applauded. Jason, who had such trouble initiating his body's movements, was carried by the audience's applause to join in. It was an action he knew like he knew how to breathe.

A few nights later a trio of jazz students came to play Spaulding's eighth-floor conference room. Muma and I, heartened by the Ralph Stanley concert, insisted that Jason hear the music despite the fact that he was already in bed when we heard about the show. A nurse helped Jason get dressed and into his wheelchair.

They were students, still a lot to learn.

Back in his room, when he was back in bed, Muma and I asked Jason if he'd liked the show.

"No."

"Oh," we said, our bubble burst, for we had been quite pleased with ourselves. "Are you glad you went?"

"Yes."

Good—he could discern between going and enjoying. And his musical taste had survived, unscathed.

Another Saturday afternoon we drove to the wheelchair-friendly movie theater on Tremont to see *Batman Begins*. In the lobby people examined Jason with bald expressions of glad-it's-not-me.

He was oblivious to the attention, but I stared back until they looked away.

He propelled himself down the hall in his wheelchair. He blew a few notes on a harmonica. His friends came in droves, and sometimes he remembered their visits after they'd left. On Monica's birthday the clan gathered for cake and ice cream in Spaulding's practice apartment, used by patients preparing to go home, which offered more space and privacy than the solarium. Jason's present for Monica came via Anne, who suggested that Jason arrive last. When Monica opened the door, she found Jason standing on his own two feet.

He was a star on the eighth floor: golden, beloved. And we felt lucky, triumphant, exhausted, exhilarated.

On the last Saturday in April we took him to a multimedia installation co-created by Lou, who was heavily involved in the local electroacoustic improvisatory scene. The piece riffed on the myth of Orpheus, the musician who follows Eurydice to Hades after she dies but breaks the one condition set by the King of the Underworld in order for Eurydice to return to life—leaving the underworld, Orpheus looks back at his beloved and loses her forever.

The next morning Jason didn't wake up. Late night, we thought. But by dinnertime he was still asleep, and his nurse, sensing something wasn't right, sent him to the ER.

23

At a red light the ambulance put on its siren and rolled through the intersection, but following in Muma's car, I had to stop. The ambulance trundled down the road like a boat heading out to sea, and I was left behind.

Time warped in the ER. Rop and I met one resident after another. Just as "I'll be back shortly" became awfully long ago, a fresh-faced doctor would bound in, hand outstretched with an introduction and the news that he or she was taking over for the previous doctor. "So," they would say, looking down at the chart, "what's going on?" And Rop and I would give Jason's medical history—all of it—all over again.

This routine lasted for hours. We'd already put in a full day, and now suddenly we were thrown into this never-ending loop. The hospital must have been running blood and urine tests, but my impression was that no one was taking charge and nothing was being done. My mind was stuck. Fear overcame me like a gas leaked from the air-conditioning vents.

In part the doctors were postponing dealing with Jason because his brain scans were upstairs in the office of Dr. Ogilvy, one of the neurosurgeons scheduled to perform the upcoming AVM surgery. These scans would provide a picture of the normal size of Jason's ventricles. From the CT scan taken when he'd come into the ER, the doctors didn't think the ventricles looked enlarged, but they couldn't be sure until they compared the scans, which couldn't happen until the office opened at 7:30 or 8:00 in the morning.

"I have a copy of the scans at home," I said to the resident at 4:00 a.m. "Should I go get them?"

"No," she said, so I didn't go. I was reluctant to leave, wanting to believe the ventricles weren't enlarged, terrified he was having seizures. Not only would seizures be bad; they would mean we'd lost the bet to take him off phenobarbital.

Throughout the night we were calling Monica and Muma with updates. "I can't think straight," I said at one point, and Fred yelled, "Marjorie, wake up! This is Jason's life!"

It was the slap I needed.

Another resident appeared in Jason's bay and introduced himself.

"Respectfully," I said, struggling to sound respectful, "I want Dr. Ogilvy. Please page him *now*."

The resident left to page the doctor—the chief of neurosurgery, the wunderkind, the bigwig, the man who wrote the book—and the nurse tending to Jason held up a gloved hand for a high-five. "I want Dr. Ogilvy!" she echoed. "All right!"

Once Dr. Ogilvy arrived, the CT scans were brought down. Chest X-ray and EEG were ordered. The doctor tapped the shunt, taking a small amount of cerebral spinal fluid to test for infection.

Jason had a slight fever, but his CSF was clear.

No seizures.

The stomach PEG came out. An NG tube was inserted through his nose.

The shunt was removed. We were back looking at the external drain.

We were back looking at the IV plumbing going into his subclavian vein.

We were back watching his numbers obsessively.

Back in a Neuro-ICU.

Back in the darkest realm of doubt, where we didn't know if Jason would be out of there in a day, a week, a month, many months. Back where we didn't know if he would be all right.

Two problems had arisen. The far end of the shunt had migrated so it was sitting on Jason's liver, blocking its opening and causing CSF to back up and enlarge his ventricles. And an infection had gotten into the shunt, the bacteria *Proprionibacterium acnes*, a "wimpy bug," according to the infectious disease doctor, but strong enough to knock Jason out.

He was put on morphine and Keppra, taken off Ritalin and amantadine. In other words, all the stimulants were out and sedatives were in. He was on three big-gun antibiotics. He slept.

"When the brain takes a hit like this, it can take one to two weeks to regain consciousness," one doctor said.

I was haunted by regret that I hadn't gone for the scans, thinking that if I had, I might have altered the diagnosis.

"You're not a doctor," a New York friend reminded me over the phone as I wandered the fruit section of a grocery store. Perhaps, given my involvement at Spaulding, I had begun to believe I was. In me was an insane desire to do this perfectly—to get an A in helping Jason, to make his story go right.

Sitting in the car in the MGH garage, I called Dr. Narayan. "A breath of calm," I wrote in my notes. He thought Jason would need a few days to recover. He thought Jason would resume his rehabilitation. He said this as if it didn't occur to him to think that Jason wouldn't.

May 4. We joke more, laugh harder in these emergency situations.

Again our routine shifted. New parking lot. New coffee shop. New protocol for the impressive and relatively new Neuro-ICU, which required being buzzed through the door by telephone.

The nurses told me about the flasher and the nun who'd shared a room. The nurses didn't worry because, due to the nun's injury, she was cursing a blue streak. "Who the hell are you?" she said when the doctor walked in.

Jason was put back on Ritalin and amantadine. He started communicating with blinks again. He remembered that.

May 5. I can't read his expression. I don't want to assume. I hope he's okay in there.

To prevent contractures, the physical therapist ordered casts for his legs and arms. The casting technician, who was also a minister, told me he'd "raised some hell" when he was young. He'd dodged the draft by sending change-of-address notices until the army caught up. He returned from Vietnam unchanged. "Are you coming to church with me?" his wife would ask, and he would reply with a long drawn-out "No." But he came up against himself, and one day he prayed for help. Within a week he quit smoking, stopped swearing, finally went to church with his wife. During the sermon he fell asleep. When the collection basket was passed around, he reached in his pocket and pulled out one of the two bills there. The minister looked at the twenty-dollar bill in the basket, but the man said, "I've been taking from the Lord for so long—He's got to take that money from me."

The man told this story openly, with humility, sharing his faith. He gave me hope.

Morning and night I was saying my prayers, but fear coated my jumbled thoughts. Afternoons, Lila and I walked in the Fells, a huge woodsy state park, and I cried and cried, feeling enraged, crushed, a wretched sadness.

May 8. Slow days. Minimal response. There isn't much to do, which drives a person nuts and allows way too much time for worrying about the unpredictable future.

May 9. What a ridiculous week. In the midst of it, I heard God. It was right after I found a parking place. I know how that sounds. I was listening to a radio broadcast of the Unitarian service. They were playing hymns I had sung in school. I knew the words. The pastor asked us to say "Lord, hear our prayer" every time she said a certain cue. I was shouting "Lord, hear our prayer" at the top of my lungs. Then she, and we, said the Lord's Prayer and I said it again and again, a mantra, as usual my tongue twisting at "not into temptation." It was then I heard a voice. I don't remember the words, but the point was: Do not doubt that I am here.

I didn't take this as a message from God that Jason would be all right. I took it as a reminder. I was not Christian. But my spirituality often used Christian words, like *God*, to carry the feeling inside me, which was, that day, *Please help.* Help Jason first but also help me and my parents and Monica and her family. We were buckling. Jason's admittance to the Neuro-ICU had coincided with other family members' medical problems. The stress was like an environmental condition, like increased barometric pressure before a thunderstorm.

The drain came out. A new shunt went in.

Stable, he moved out of the Neuro-ICU to the Neuro unit.

Again, we stuck pictures of friends and family to the walls. Because why not, we pinned the tiny sack with little stones to his pillow, which someone had blessed with healing properties.

"What did he used to do?" a nurse asked, looking at Jason as if he lay not in a bed but a coffin.

"He *is* a musician," I said, insisting on the present tense. "He plays guitar and he sings."

"He sings?" the nurse said. "We had a patient who sang Irish music. Her family brought in her CD. It was *eerie* hearing her voice. She was lying there, just like Jason. She recovered. Don't know if she ever sang again."

"Jason was so vocal before this week," I said. "I believe if he wants to sing again, he will."

"It's a goal," the nurse said doubtfully.

"Do they think he's going to pull out of this?" another nurse asked.

This was unacceptable, Monica told the nurse manager in no uncertain terms. One of the nurses was replaced. As when we had fired Dr. Dear, we worried that criticizing the nurses would jeopardize his care. But even now, depleted, wrenched, we insisted that the people working with him treat him like a living, breathing human being. When the new nurse assigned to Jason suggested to Rop and me that we go on a Duck Boat tour of Boston Harbor, we nodded and said nothing in reply.

Jason's roommate was a mailman, about sixty years old.

"He does most of his eating in the morning," said the woman with him.

The mailman had cancer. "Look at that." He was reading the newspaper. "Decrease of cancer risk from the UV rays. After all these years of telling us to wear sunblock."

"Ain't it always the way," the woman said. "I never wear sunblock. Except after I get burned. You watch Maury?"

"I'd rather watch Jerry."

They were days of heavy rain, days of not flipping out when I wanted to flip out, days when the thinnest film separated me from a breakdown. The only option was to take the next step forward. Take a deep breath and look at the real day and figure out my immediate next action. Nights I escaped into movies, mainly military movies: *Patton, A Bridge Too Far, The Bridge on the River Kwai*. Stories of mission and collective effort were the only stories I wanted to be told.

May 20. I am Patton *and* the soldier with the frayed nerves.

May 22. J said, "Hi Moe," when I came in.

The stomach PEG went back in, the last medical procedure before Jason could return to Spaulding. Now MGH's physiatrist had to recommend that Jason receive intensive rehab at Spaulding; the case manager had to relay this information to Spaulding; Spaulding had to tell Mass Health it would take Jason because Jason would benefit from Spaulding; Mass Health had to agree (a high hurdle: its guidelines favored physical progress over cognitive improvement); Jason had to tolerate the stomach PEG; then, once these pieces were in place, a bed had to open up.

On May 24 I woke up angry and saw that I was angry.
"God," I said, "help. How can I not be angry?"
I read some psalms. I looked in the Big Book for advice on anger. I got on my knees and prayed. I asked for loving-kindness. Later that day we got word that Jason had been approved to return to Spaulding.
I did not think that my prayer had caused the approval. I was only relieved. Even as I was praying, reading, trying to let go, I was full of doubt. But I had no other choice. I had to deal with the anger somehow. It was an anger that felt greater than a human emotion. It was like a sandstorm. I sought refuge in the only shelter I could see.
"We're all pulling for him," said one of the doctors as we were leaving, and I heard these words as if they were spoken by everyone, everywhere, in the whole world.

24

We arrived back at Spaulding the day before Jason's thirty-fifth birthday, all of us in bad shape. Rop snapped at a nurse. Muma was manic. Jason was coughing. Rashes covered his body. His arms shook wildly. "Is he having a seizure?" the wife of his new roommate asked, innocent to our history with that question. My volcanic frustration was barely disguised when I answered no. Not seizures, but what? Was the shaking his attempt to initiate movement or misfired signals in his brain? Or medication? Why was he so unresponsive?

May 29. How can I say it except I love Jason so much and the desire to have him regain his health consumes every part of me. There are moments when it feels he will slip out of our grasp. Simultaneously, I simply believe he will recover.

Notes in my journal shortened. I couldn't write much more than excuses for writing so little. The misery was too difficult to record.

He had been a prize patient. Now he was—who knew? Even the staff was rattled.

"The shaking really freaked me out," a nurse acknowledged.

"Gee," one therapist said, "he's back at square one."

E. coli was detected in his urine, and he was put on antibiotics.

A week after Jason's return, a former Spaulding patient dropped in to say hello to the people who had worked with him. We had heard about Noah because he and Jason were about the same age and Noah's family had been similarly involved in his recovery. His sister, Kate, had moved to Boston to help him—she was the one whose name Margaret had transferred to me.

Noah had been driving his car when a sudden snowstorm swept in. He'd collided with an oncoming vehicle. So quickly told, such lasting consequences. He was at Spaulding for eleven months. He didn't talk for nine of them. Worse than Jason, we'd heard.

And yet here stood a vibrant articulate man, not only talking and walking but holding several conversations at once, describing the 5K race he'd run last week, jogging up and down the corridor so Anne could see how an ankle problem had resolved. I watched her watch him with her expert eye.

When Margaret called me by his sister's name, I had chalked it up to a mistake. But now, meeting Noah and Kate, the so-called mistake seemed prescient. The resemblances between our families, between Jason and Noah and Kate and me, made me think we were meeting our doppelgängers. Here was Jason's potential future.

Everyone was talking about Noah. People were crying with happiness.

"It's God's doing," said a nurse's aide.

"And hard work," I insisted.

"But it is up to Him," another aide replied. "If you are *breathing* after something like that, it is God."

June 7. I feel ferocious, just totally bloodthirsty, for yes. For his coming home. For this time. For okay, life is suffering, life is hard and gets harder, and we are made of durable stuff that won't take no for an answer, that will not accept anything other than a full recovery to a full independent life. Thank God for Monica, Muma, and Rop: absolute believers in this goal.

Jason regained lost ground, in three weeks covering the work of his previous three months at Spaulding. With medication stabilized and regular therapy resumed, the shaking abated. Quiet, underweight, unsteady, nevertheless he advanced from the Atlas Walker to walking freely while supported by two people, one on either side. Choosing his meals from a menu became daily routine. He ate breakfast with other patients in the dining room. He joined a balance practice group that kicked and tossed foam or rubber balls back and forth with a spotter standing behind. Some PT sessions he and Anne and I rode around the little riverside park on low recumbent bicycles.

"Who is the problem?" we asked.

"Moe," he replied, with quivering lips.

"I'm glad you're here," he said when I arrived one morning.

His arm came up on my shoulder as I embraced him.

"That's nice," he said when I relayed Ben Rubin's I-miss-you voice mail message. "Bass," he said when I asked what Ben played.

"I love you too," he said.

"So, Moe," he began, as he always had.

"Ipso," he said for the " ___ facto" crossword puzzle clue.

"I feel out of it," he said, and we cheered that he could differentiate feeling out of it from normal.

Examining his fingers, whose contractures were, despite dozens of casts and splints, still very severe, he asked, "Am I going to be able to play again?" The heartbreaking question at least signaled that he was assembling the big picture.

Jason would come home from Spaulding—but what home? Monica, Lou, and Jane found an apartment for sale near Inman Square, a three-bedroom with a backyard and a finished basement that could be Jason's studio. Walking Lila past Lou and Jane's house one afternoon, I stopped to chat with Jane, who was in an upstairs window.

"What are you guys up to?" I asked.

"Liquidating," she replied.

The plan for now was for me to live with Jason, with Ellie and Monica staying with her parents and Muma and Rop continuing their alternating commutes from New York. In June we left the Harvard Street apartment and I moved out of my Brooklyn studio. No more forwarded mail, no more shaking down the subletter for utility bill reimbursement. I was sleeping in my own bed again, taking for my room half of the basement, which, with its pearl-colored carpet and sea-blue walls, felt like a cove. Stacks of cardboard boxes shared the space with me: Jason's gear and equipment; boxes yet unpacked brought from the storage unit in Newton; my own unneeded belongings, like pots and pans, winter clothes, books. My bedroom was carved from a surrounding temporariness.

The apartment, with a large central kitchen, living room, and dining room, took up the first floor of a new building that was being constructed on an empty lot adjacent to a social club whose members did not like losing their off-street parking. When I moved in, the building's two other units were not finished, the driveway and backyard were dirt, and there were confusions and delays with the electricity and phone companies—all fine. Living on a construction site matched the rest of my life.

Even as we arranged furniture and unpacked plates and dishes and silverware, we were outfitting the apartment with a shower bench, raised toilet seat, bed rails.

Jason was coming home.

In late July a beam of protons zapped the AVM. For the surgery Jason wore a mask of plastic like the white skirt of a badminton birdie that had been molded to fit his face and snapped to the underside of the table on which he lay. The mask's mouthpiece further ensured that his head was immobile. Using an MRI as a map and ball bearings embedded in his skull as markers, technicians aligned the three-story-high atom splitter to target the AVM.

Because children sometimes lay under the giant machine, stuffed monkeys with Velcro paws hung from some of its white metal limbs. The surgery lasted forty-five minutes. In the crowded waiting room exotic fish swam in a tank, and a woman played a harp. Afterward we returned to Spaulding. Later that day Jason ate dinner.

"What are you thinking about?" I asked one quiet afternoon.

"My body," he replied.

"In what way?"

"I want it to move, but it won't do what I ask."

And yet it could. He'd wanted to shift positions, but a pillow behind his back was preventing him. I took away the pillow, lowered the bed, and he was able, with just a little help from me, to roll onto his other side.

That night I dreamed Jason and I were in an empty house. He made a recording on the answering machine, which I listened to twice. "Isn't it funny," he said on the tape, "that we think we have a will of our own, when a person can ask his body to move and it won't?"

Give up your idea of a will, I thought when I awoke.

We passed the one-year anniversary of his bleed preparing for his homecoming. Speaking, eating, walking, biking, shaving, cracking jokes, getting dressed, using the bathroom—in performing these activities at all, he had far surpassed the expectations of his doctors, with the notable exception of Dr. Narayan.

Had we thwarted fate? Or was he fated to be a phoenix reborn from the ashes of his former self?

Unchecked and unchallenged, standard medical care and insurance would not have given him the recovery he had thus far achieved.

We had intervened. And yet we were answering something that was years in the making—our love for who he was.

The one corporeal piece that decided everything none but an oracle could have known: his injury, though complicated, nevertheless allowed for recovery. The possibility for mending existed.

If you are breathing after something like that, it is God.

Alone, he could not have done it.

If his motivation has been knocked out, we will provide surrogate motivation until his returns.

But we could not have been more than surrogates. Determination, as much as potential, had to be there. Knowing him, we'd bet it was. Then, even in his most minute actions, we saw it was.

The most advanced technology. The ancient laying on of hands. And desire in the deepest part of him.

Without us he could not have exercised the free will to get well. He would have been denied that choice. And yet we fought to give him that choice precisely because of the person he had worked so hard throughout his life to be.

Lying in his bed, he thought he could not move his body. But the obstacle had proved temporary, illusory. He had far more of a will than he'd concluded, though it was a will that existed in the outer boundaries of personhood—belonging not entirely to him nor to those around him, playing somewhere on the border of body and spirit, a conduit to the divine cosmos, at once greater than, other than, no more than all of us.

25

A year and a week after the bleed, he came home.

Cautious, still seeing double, his body stiff and thin, balance wavering, with one of us on either side, holding him, guiding him, he walked through the front door.

I'd driven away from Spaulding with Jason beside me in the passenger seat. What if this was the story? He survived a brain hemorrhage, meningitis, coma, seizures, then died in a car crash while leaving the hospital.

But we had arrived safely. Maybe like this we could make our way, moment of fear followed by moment of victory.

He sank into the blue couch, winded by the walk from the car. Monica brought him his wedding ring, which, early on, she'd been advised to take for safekeeping.

"Will you marry me?" she said, an impish glee in her voice, and he replied earnestly, "Yes."

It wouldn't slide on his ring finger—still too bent—so she put it on his right hand.

Then she found a pair of scissors and cut the red and white hospital bracelet from his wrist.

He was no longer a patient.

26

In the beginning I saw Jason at the hospital and went home to my Brooklyn studio. Then I spent my days with Jason and slept in an apartment I shared with my parents. Now I was submerged. No more visitors' hours. No more leaving at night, trusting he was in the hands of good, experienced licensed professionals. Now the responsibility for all his care, all the time, fell on us.

In the hospital nurses took medications from a cart in the hall stocked by the pharmacy. Nurse's aides helped him shower and dress and changed his sheets. Therapists set goals and assignments. The cafeteria made meals. The janitor emptied the garbage. The social worker communicated with Mass Health. After twelve hours the next shift arrived. Now we played all these roles. Grueling physical labor coincided with mental overload.

"It's like we suddenly have to learn how to fly an airplane," Monica said.

There wasn't time in the day to second-guess our decision. The lack of choice was one less thing to think about, and our unquestioned commitment yielded a requisite confidence. We were doing this because we believed we *could* do this. And that he could. By a logic both natural and stunning, I chose Inman Pharmacy, the closest drugstore, for Jason's prescriptions because, I reasoned, one day Jason would fill his prescriptions himself. Not yet. Not soon. But why wouldn't his palpable momentum carry him to that day?

But beneath my confidence ran the fear that the AVM would rebleed, the shunt would malfunction, he would trip, he would choke, and we would be helpless. In the hospital, in an emergency, we could push a button and someone would come to our aid. No more button now.

Our inexperience loomed before us, but we had one particular skill, honed over the previous fifty-three weeks. We knew how to watch Jason. Vigilance was our stock-in-trade. A piece of me was ever tuned to him, and the patchwork sentinel made of my parents, Monica, and me convinced me that any disaster would not go unnoticed.

For his every movement—sitting down, standing up, standing in place, taking even one step—at least one of us was with him. Frail and imbalanced, barely and irregularly able to start actions and conversations, even to express hunger or fatigue, he could stall out halfway through a meal, fork in hand, inert. Then we hovered, waiting, wondering—should we intervene so he wouldn't get discouraged or go hungry, or let him go at his own slow pace? Sometimes we tapped his elbow and his arm would reignite and the food would reach his mouth. Other times he needed someone to feed him. As we moved with him, so we had to think for him. Except for when he was sound asleep, we were always working.

Afternoons Jason would nap, and my parents and I would crash too, hard, no choice but to give way to a crushing fatigue from whose oblivion I would awaken to different light, later in the day.

Once, at Spaulding, he'd gotten up around midnight, setting off his bed alarm. Nurses had found him standing beside his roommate, a teenage boy who cried in a high moan.

"I wanted to see if he needed help," Jason had explained.

That's so Jason, we'd said proudly when we'd heard this. Now we worried that, unaware of his dodgy balance, he would try to stand or walk and fall. He had fallen before, at St. Vincent's. Even with bed rails, a bed alarm, and a monitor so I could hear him from downstairs, we checked on him around one in the morning. Potential regret—that tomorrow I would learn there'd been a problem and I hadn't gotten up—never failed to prod my tired body out of bed.

Sometimes his catheter had leaked and his sheets needed to be changed, which we'd learned how to do with him in the bed, and we would fix the catheter and change him into clean pajamas. These were Texas catheters, like a condom with an opening at the far end, which attached to a tube that ran to a urine bag. Putting a catheter on my brother was awkward and strange, but I aimed for a low-key, no-fuss approach. Just another of a thousand interactions.

Jason's first afternoon home I stood in his bedroom holding the lid to a jar of "catheter cement," to which was attached a little brush from which dripped the glue.

"I never use the stuff," said the personal care attendant beside me, a large woman who in a few days would quit, saying the atmosphere was too claustrophobic—an honest review.

Mass Health was paying for fifty-five hours per week of PCA help. Monica, who was overseeing schedules, timesheets, and payroll, had posted job listings, interviewed candidates, hired a handful, then fired some, like the German who insisted on being barefoot. Eventually we would find the obvious solution in two strong, lovely, loving aides from Spaulding—Diane, a tart-tongued Bostonian, and sweet Addis, originally from Ethiopia—but in Jason's first days home the apartment was crowded with too many PCAs, people we didn't know, who didn't know us, like this woman now who was watching me, breathing down my neck.

I put the catheter on as I'd been taught at Spaulding. The unforgiving cement made a sticky mess of the catheter while also sealing in some pubic hair.

"Get some scissors," said the PCA.

"Scissors?"

"How else are you going to get this off?"

Every part of me cringed. Even my internal organs seemed to shrink. Could I entrust Jason to this woman? She was a licensed nurse. But I didn't know her. My parents were asleep. There was no one to consult. The catheter had to come off. Far outside the safety of the hospital, far from standards and protocols, I handed a stranger the scissors, and she fixed the situation.

27

The injury had begun with blood gushing from a broken vessel, seeping into crevices of Jason's brain, damaging whatever it touched, damming his aqueduct of Sylvius—the path of water through the forest, in my rough translation. His recovery was like hacking through that forest, crawling under downed trees, groping in darkness; no map, only the forest as guide to the swamps, the loops—sometimes a glade.

At dinner on his third night home, Jason picked up a knife to cut his food. Behind this simple act stretched a path, winding, bending, doubling back, lost, now found again, through hospitals, medications, exercises, casts, and splints, through his efforts and ours and those of the doctors and therapists, through the prayers and kindnesses of friends and family and the village of Dr. Narayan's mother-in-law. The path that led to his picking up the knife spontaneously, as if it were nothing to do so, was a path through thick forest ending at an emerald pool surrounded by majestic redwoods.

We had no way of knowing what was going to work, what would come easily, which path led where. The forest was full of dead ends. A pager service sent Jason twice-daily texts on his cell phone—

MEDICINE—so, ideally, instead of us handing him the pills and water at noon and four, he would get them himself. But often he was away from his phone or saw the text and then, distracted, forgot about it. Switching activities abruptly was perhaps too great a challenge, as was forming a plan to get a glass, fill it with water, get the medicine, and take it.

We tried rock climbing in Spaulding's outdoor adaptive sports program. I thought it would lengthen his tight muscles, but the weight on his contracted finger joints caused excruciating pain. Worse, he wasn't very vocal—few words in a soft monotone—and only after an hour of climbing, when the pain had become unbearable, could he say he wanted to stop. Having championed the rock climbing idea, I felt responsible and miserable, though not, I knew, as miserable as he had felt doing it.

Engaged in the usual triumvirate of therapies in Spaulding's outpatient division, Jason was assigned a speech therapist, young and inexperienced, who presented one standardized worksheet after another. Bored, Jason nodded off. First Dr. Dear, then the MGH nurse, now the speech therapist—it never got easier to say "This isn't working" without worrying that requesting a change would give us a bad reputation. The switch was worth our discomfort. Peter, the second speech therapist, tailored the treatment to Jason, whose first assignment was to write out the lyrics to two songs. He chose one he'd written, "Dixie," and a favorite, Warren Zevon's "Poor Poor Pitiful Me." "What do these songs mean to you?" Peter asked at their next session. "What inspired 'Dixie?'" The point was to get Jason writing and speaking again, but with the exercise grounded in something he loved, appropriately the line blurred between therapy and two guys discussing music.

A week after he came home, Muma, Jason, and I set out to see *Revenge of the Sith* at the Harvard Square Cinema, but when we arrived, the movie had already started.

"The paper always screws up the times," said the kid in the box office.

Muma helped Jason into the car while I loaded the wheelchair, then we raced over to the Fresh Pond Mall, but its listing was also wrong. The last screening was yesterday.

Should we head home, try again tomorrow?

There was one more possibility. If we hurried, we might miss the previews but we'd make the movie. Muma guided Jason into the passenger seat as I broke down the wheelchair.

At the Somerville Theatre the end credits were rolling. The next screening wouldn't start for forty-five minutes. I ran across the street for ice cream, and as we sat, waiting, Jason recalled that he had performed here several times, for the movie theater was also a music venue. It was an old vaudeville house, with ornate but faded fixtures and mouldings and a stage of well-worn wood that inspired Muma to say she felt like doing a tap-dance.

"No one's stopping you," Jason said dryly.

In chasing down the movie, Muma and I were operating, as did Rop and Monica, according to a mind-set that said, Go all the way all the time. It was backbreaking, but how else would we find out what worked? How else would Jason reconnect impulse with action, desire with acquisition?

He fell asleep. The next day he wouldn't remember the movie. But our efforts earned a surprise reward. That night, going home, he got in the car differently. He'd been using a two-step procedure—lower into the passenger seat with someone spotting, then swivel to face forward. Leaving Somerville, Jason slid into the car elegantly, normally, ducking his head, extending his left leg as he sank into the seat, bringing his right leg in as he pulled the door closed. The prize, ours as much as his, propelled us forward, knowing that our instincts were right, our toil worthwhile. The more he ventured into the world, the more he responded to it.

Mornings we played Connect 4 for fine motor skills, Scattergories for word retrieval. "You share this with someone you care about," he said for *umbrella*, "especially in bad weather."

Arriving at Spaulding one afternoon, I helped Jason out of the car as Rop unfolded the wheelchair.

"You want to walk or ride?" I asked, meaning, do you want to walk or ride *to the curb*, after which I figured he'd go in the wheelchair.

"Walk." He turned and called out, "I don't need it."

Rop looked at me, wondering if he'd heard correctly.

I shrugged, baffled.

He never used the wheelchair again.

If asked he could say that he'd had a bleed in his head, but the details lay beyond his grasp. At the end of the day he might remember some of what he'd done, but most of it was like a waterfall: over the cliff and gone. He went where we took him, ate food put before him. Monica brought Ellie over daily, but Jason didn't register who the baby was. She appeared before him the way everything else did: there, gone, forgotten.

The offer of a free Palm Pilot enticed us to enroll Jason in a study on short-term memory. The Palm Pilot sent him reminders and gave him his schedule, but more significant, once synced with his computer, it held phone numbers for his friends, whom he started calling because he was better able to converse on the phone than in person, although sometimes he called people six or seven times in a day, the earlier conversations having evaporated from his mind.

Down by the Charles River one afternoon, we stopped to pet a chocolate lab. "What a great dog," I said as the dog and his owner walked away.

"What dog?" Jason asked.

And yet. Something in him said "Walk." Slid into the car. Picked up the knife. Something in him was accepting the thousands of challenges presented by ordinary daily life.

"How long is it going to take me to get over this?" he asked Dr. Chae at his first checkup, about a month after coming home.

"I can't give you a finite number," replied Dr. Chae. "But the fact that you're asking is an excellent sign."

28

August 21. Oh, Lord! For the day when I am again in my own home, wherever it may be.

Because I was living with Jason full-time, was the person constantly with him, I emerged as the manager of his schedule, refiller of his prescriptions, restocker of supplies, communicator with doctors. Rop or Muma was with me for the daily hands-on work, and Monica, as much as possible while also taking care of Ellie, but I was the point person, a role I took on willingly, feeling capable, grateful even, for an outlet for my fanatic pursuit of Jason's recovery. But sometimes I thought my head would explode.

Out of the blue Mass Health would not cover prescriptions without "prior authorization," and I bounced between pharmacy, primary care physician, Dr. Chae, and Mass Health, my frustration merging with a stubborn determination to win this battle, to prove—to no one but myself—that I would not retreat until this latest obstacle was overcome. Meanwhile, Jason needed compression socks to counteract swelling in his feet and lamb's wool so armrests would not rub raw his delicate skin; he needed to be tested for nerve damage on his left foot, which dropped, and to be fitted for a brace to correct the drop. His energy was low—a possible urinary tract infection? Schedule an appointment—yes, UTI—back to the pharmacy for Bactrim. Each day was like running a long-distance cross-country course , never a chance to stop, only the occasional opportunity to slow to a jog. Gradually, the arduous course became familiar—or the arduousness of the course came to be expected in my back and arm muscles and behind my eyes, where exhaustion pulled.

Jason's recovery was tremendous but clearly defined work. The rest of my situation was more complicated. Accustomed to living on my own, now it was like I lived in Grand Central. And it wasn't as though my parents and I were sharing an apartment but going to separate jobs. We were together in this project, all of us totally dedicated, none of us a professional doctor or nurse or PCA. It had been seventeen years since our family had split up. To come together now was to find that the edges of the pieces had roughened. We didn't fit the way we used to. There were flare-ups, too, between Monica and me. The setup was inherently awkward. My parents and I were living with Jason in an apartment that belonged to him and Monica, using their furniture and kitchenware, while Monica and Ellie lived with her parents. We were not guests; we were not quite at home. Even though everyone understood and no one could see an alternative, we were a strained group.

There was no self-pity. The Crigler Family talent at holding back and stifling feelings—not a fabulous trait in general—served us well. We didn't want minor tensions to destroy the operation. We didn't want Jason to feel guilty. We all chose to do this. No one thought it would be easy. To this communally difficult situation each of us brought liabilities but also talents. We were all neurotic, manic control freaks with deep reserves of affection and strength and endurance. We had never done anything like this before. We couldn't have done it and done it *right*.

September 8. I guess this is a stressful situation. I forget sometimes.

Near the end of my freshman year at Stanford I injured my back, nearly slipping a disk, and a doctor told me that if I didn't want surgery I'd better start swimming. Monday to Friday at noon I worked out with the Masters swim team, open to any students, faculty, or alumni. That I had never swum competitively didn't bother the coaches, who trained the school's swim teams and sometimes the U.S. Olympic teams. They put me in a slow lane and taught me technique, how to breathe effectively, how to do a proper flip turn. Swimming saved my back and, unexpectedly, brought some relief to my mind as well.

Now, hoping swimming might relieve the constant strain in my neck and shoulders, I joined the Masters team at Cambridge War Memorial Pool, where everything was cement or metal and Band-Aids and hairbands littered the deep end. Excessive chlorine—the pool was attached to a high school—made my throat sore and stuffed up my nose. Only a dozen people made up the team. Our coach was a librarian. Twice a week, for an hour and a half, my only thoughts were breathing and form and how many laps.

September 15. Started swimming the longer workouts. So much energy to burn.

Though tired, I was revving high, somehow both exhausted and productive. I drank a lot of coffee and kept going. This approach was unsustainable, but the situation was temporary. The end date was impossible to predict, but we would know it when we saw it.

Halfway through the Masters practice, the high school girls' synchronized swim team started theirs. On land they moved their arms as they would later move their legs. Resting between sets, I would hear them outline their choreography—*that head thingie, then la-la-la*—and then Queen or Michael Jackson or ABBA would be piped underwater. Later, in the locker room, bundling up against the cold night, I'd see the varsity team rehearsing, their arm dances

155

interspersed with gossip about who liked whom and the party at the house of a girl from another school whose parents were *total hippies* and had a room full of pot plants. The ease with which the girls interacted was inaccessible to me, as if the window that had descended into my life on August 5, separating me from the rest of the world, were still in place. I had become so accustomed to it that only now, as I stepped back into a normal activity, did I feel it again.

Some late afternoons I went to Café Pamplona for cappuccino and to eavesdrop on conversations. In the old Cambridge coffee-house I imagined heated defenses of Trotsky but instead heard about trips to Alaska:

"Is it threaded with creeks?"

"No, it's spotted with lakes."

By the time I returned home after Masters, the skin around my eyes still dented from my goggles, Rop would have helped Jason into bed, and I would slip downstairs.

My Brooklyn studio had been about the same square footage as the space I now occupied in the half of the basement with the window and glass door looking onto a stairwell that led up to the backyard. Bed, dresser, two desks, a chair, a bookshelf, kitchen table, two stools: the sum total of my furniture. Sometimes I opened one of the boxes stacked in the corner, looking for a particular book, say, or scarf, and felt like I was peering into another world. To glimpse the artifacts of my old familiar life was to remember fully for a fleeting moment a person I once knew well. I was divided, partially on hold. Here there wasn't room for all of me.

At Family Strategies, a Spaulding class in which families and survivors talked about challenges at home, the wife of an elderly man said that since his stroke she'd had no life. Every minute of every day she took care of him. One hour per week a relative relieved her. Hiring a PCA would mean training the PCA—one more job for the wife.

"I'm a prisoner," she said plainly.

I recognized myself in the facts of her story, though I did not feel imprisoned. My situation was demanding, sometimes frustrating, but it was one I had chosen and it was impermanent. Monica and Jason would not live apart forever, and I had no illusion that I would spend the rest of my life as Jason's aide. I had turned down a few TV production job offers, but I was being paid some of the Mass Health PCA money. I'd joined Grub Street, a Boston writers' group, where I was making new friends. I was writing stories, reading them at open mike nights, submitting them for publication.

If the loneliness of my path was acute, I never doubted what I was doing. Parts of adulthood had baffled me—how to write and make a living, why people so rarely took risks, whether to salt eggplant before cooking it—but contributing to Jason's recovery was something my prior years had prepared me for, one of the few moments in grown-up life that was directly in line with the purpose of all that had come before. The specifics of brain injury and medicine had had to be learned, but opting to participate was a question long since settled. Literature had given me countless tales of loyalty and gambles. A middle-class upbringing and rigorous schools had taught me to work. The joy of my childhood, followed by the pain of my parents' breakup, had shown me that I could decide my role in this family; the shape of our story depended partly on me. My daily struggles—this was the work of it. This was Odysseus battling gods and monsters for ten years to get home to Penelope. This was Beowulf killing the demon Grendel. If only all of life's decisions could be as simple as choosing to help someone I loved.

But—this much help? In this deep?

That's right.

This much. This deep.

Like stone yielding a sculpture, the other half of the basement was transforming from a lump of boxes and gear into a studio. Rop, Monica, and I assembled Jason's desk and computer, built bookshelves, mounted guitar hooks on the wall. Jason was with us, but often after opening a box, he would discover something—a notebook, a photo album—and fall into the find, hunched over, absorbed, lost in it. He hadn't packed any of this, after all. He had walked out of their Douglass Street apartment to play a gig thinking he'd return later that night.

He seemed to be retracing earlier times, as if running his fingers over a familiar cloth. Repeatedly he watched all three seasons of *The Greatest American Hero*, newly released on DVD, in which a rogue FBI agent and a high school teacher, using superpowers from an alien suit whose instruction manual has been lost, catch bad guys and save the world. When we were young and each allowed to pick one television show during the week, this was Jason's choice. (Mine was *Family Ties*.) He so loved this series, he would tape-record episodes and listen to them until the cassette wore out. Once we tried taking action shots but paid Fotomat for twenty-four pictures of a gray screen. As if I'd watched it yesterday, I could anticipate dialogue, plot twists, hokey special effects, even the incidental music. The familiarity could only have been more intense for Jason, who seemed comforted by the old stories and characters.

Pieces of our past reverberated through our present. Fridays Rop left Cambridge for New York, and Muma didn't arrive until very late, leaving Jason and me on our own for the night, as we had been for so many years while our parents played the show. In the basement we were splitting a shared room. Spaulding's outdoor sports program had an assortment of recumbent bicycles, and once a week Jason, Rop, and I, with an adaptive sports guide, rode miles down the path that ran alongside the Charles. Jason's preference, a lowrider, reminded me of his early bikes, and the rides themselves were like the rides we used to take throughout East Haddam.

Over and over he asked me about former boyfriends and classmates from grammar and high school. Where were they now? What were they doing? He ran Muma and Rop through the same interrogation. What prompted the host of the dinner party to throw baby Jason's toy giraffe in the hall? When they lived in the Village in the 1960s, why on earth didn't they go see Bob Dylan?

"We were classical musicians," they would reply. "He wasn't our scene."

The questions sprang from Jason's droll personality. But often he would perseverate, unable to move to another topic.

During the long stretches of empty time—driving to and from doctors and therapy sessions, sitting in waiting rooms—we sang. Not hymns, traditionals, show tunes, pop tunes, standards, or anything vaguely respectable but inane made-up songs, each song just half a verse repeated with variations, ad infinitum, ad nauseum. These included: "Doin' My Thing-Thing," "Goggleman," "If You Want to Know What It's Like to Be a Bon-Don (Just Ask Me)," "The Code of the Valley Girl," "Moegger the Doegger," "Muddy Moegger," "Go Moegger" (or Joegger/Mondo/Muma/Rop), "Peace and Love, Love and War," "Bossy Schwester," and "Weird Underwear" (our name for the Depends that Jason wore). Many of the songs featured a lengthy improvisation in which we tried to outwit or outlast each other. The songs were a resurrected dialect of our childhood. But also we—all of us—were together for so many hours that the supply of normal subjects ran out, leaving us with only nonsense to discuss.

To gain weight, he was referred to a nutritionist, whose suggestions included foods with fat, like nuts, avocados, eggs.

"So," Jason said slyly, "I should eat ice cream?"

"Ice cream is okay," the nutritionist allowed.

"I *should* eat it, then?"

He called ice cream *bombo*. His pager was *Percy*. His leg brace was *Bruce*. The foam roller for back exercises was *Fontainebleau*. A bowl of ice cream with two flavors was *combo-bombo*, which we usually had after dinner, settling into the couch for an episode of *Star Trek: Voyager*, in which the USS Voyager and its crew are sucked into the Delta Quadrant of the universe, seventy thousand light-years from home. Through the fall and winter of 2005–2006 we watched all seven seasons, start to finish, escaping into tales of the Maquis, Captain Janeway, and Species 8472. What was the story of *Voyager* but our story? A valiant crew, determined to reach home, is beset by detours, enemies, battles, and setbacks. When would we arrive? Where would we be next week? Impossible to say.

October 16. Dreamed Jay started singing, dancing, prancing, with a hat on his head and a determined expression like, I can do it. I know how.

"I'm so tired of this," he said.

We wanted to give him a break from his body and mind—or at least find a way to fool his mind into forgetting his body's limitations.

Spaulding's modest swim therapy program allowed Jason to swap one of his PT sessions for a session in the pool. At the Newton Marriott Hotel, past the revolving door with the floral arrangement in its hub, past the shiny polished lobby, down two floors, past the Pilgrim Suite, at the end of a narrow hall, the little pool awaited us.

We were always late, Rop and Jason and me, always racing down the Pike, seagulls screaming bloody murder over the railroad tracks.

Hotel guests also used the pool, so as Jason and the PT float-walked from one end to the other or rode imaginary bikes, a woman might be doing laps along the side or kids might be jumping in, getting out, jumping in again. Soon I was getting in, too, so after his session he could stay in the water. Then we'd sit in the hot tub, almost always with a local fellow, a regular, a large chatty man with a Salvador Dali mustache. Once, while I was waiting for Jason and Rop to emerge from the locker room, Salvador Dali complimented me for helping my "special needs" brother, and I could feel the explanation line up, ready to be spoken, but instead I said thanks and turned away, realizing he was like someone looking at a photo of an arrow launched from a bow who thinks the arrow will suspend in midair forever, when the truth is that the arrow is in motion, shooting forward fast.

In the pool Jason would float on his back, my hand under him for support. He seemed relaxed then, released, and I would test how little effort was needed to hold him up.

Sometimes I could keep him afloat with no more than my pinkie.

29

"What are you thinking about?" I asked. We were sitting at the table after breakfast.

"Leaves and trees," he said. "Being outside."

As we protected him physically, so we tried to protect him from thinking *I can't*.

With nothing on the schedule until afternoon, Monica and Ellie met Jason, Rop, and me at the Fells, the large wooded wilderness twenty minutes north of Cambridge, where I often hiked with Lila. Under red and yellow leaves we walked about an eighth of a mile. Then he was winded. We rested on a stone wall, then turned back.

In pictures from that day Jason wears a searching expression. He doesn't smile. His face is thin. He seems a shrunken version of himself. His nose veers to the right, from where the NG tube pulled it. His neck stretches forward, reshaped after months of being propped up by too many pillows. In some of the pictures, under his glasses, he wears an eye patch.

The hemorrhage had knocked Jason's eyes out of alignment. Primarily, his left eye turned down. The double images appeared vertically, a ghost hovering above or below the real thing. Not only had nerves controlling his eye muscles been damaged by the torrent of leaking blood, but over the past year his brain had accepted the strabismus and now expected to perceive two images. Surgery would work best, would perhaps *only* work, after the eye muscles had been strengthened and his mind had been retaught to see the world in one image, no ghosts.

The first fix suggested by Varsha, his OT, was temporary and gentle: a strip of Scotch tape on the lower third of his eyeglass lens, to encourage the left eye to look up. Then Rop thought of the eye patch, which exchanged depth perception for a single image. To avoid over- or underworking either eye, we switched the patch every hour. Immediately, Jason's demeanor shifted. No longer suspicious of what was real and what ghost, he became less hesitant, reaching for his mug of tea without needing his fingertips to tell him which mug, walking up stairs without overshooting each step. But the patch was not a long-term solution—at the pool he walked into a glass door, his soft hands colliding with the handle, his newfound confidence shattered—and we began to research vision specialists and eye surgeons.

And orthodontists. His teeth looked like they belonged to a nineteenth-century street peddler, some falling in, others crowded out. "They must have been like that before the bleed," a New York doctor had insisted. "He had braces!" we'd replied. "His teeth were perfect!"

The elderly orthodontist, who came recommended, bent over Jason's mouth. After a moment he sighed. "Extensive damage," he dictated to a resident. "Surgery." Another long sigh. "Extraction." Sigh. "Braces." Sigh. The doctor seemed overwhelmed by the degree of destruction, a feeling he offered us free of charge. "You need to decide," he said, "whether it's worth it to Jason to undergo this much mouth work."

You're goddamn right it's worth it, and you can ask Jason, who's sitting right here, I wanted to say but didn't.

With crooked teeth would he smile less, talk less? Would he hold back, embarrassed? Left as they were, his teeth would be harder to clean, could harbor infections. By *worth* did the doctor refer to the length of treatment or its financial cost? In excluding Jason from the conversation, the doctor clearly believed Jason's mind was as crumpled as his mouth. Was he suggesting some people weren't *worth* good teeth?

A second opinion confirmed the diagnosis. Contractures had narrowed Jason's palate and squeezed his teeth, and not eating for so many months had warped his bite, that is, how his teeth fit together. The remedy existed, but it would be long and intricate—palate expansion surgery, teeth extraction, braces. Mass Health would cover the surgery. Thanks to the benefit concerts, Monica and Jason had the seven thousand dollars needed for the rest, but I could imagine not having the money, no choice but to accept the damage as permanent. I imagined it would feel like leaving part of Jason behind.

When Jason was in the ICUs, even well into rehab, he couldn't inform us of his double vision. Even if he had, the eye problems would have taken a back seat to his survival. We had seen his teeth rearrange, but as long as he wasn't eating, they were a lower priority than keeping him alive or figuring out how to rouse him. Until recently he hadn't been stable enough to even consider palate surgery or braces. The proton beam radiation, to treat the AVM, had been the most important surgery, and he hadn't been ready for that until July; two weeks later he'd come home. Now we were dealing with problems that, understandably, had fallen outside the hospitals' scope. Still, it was odd that tackling these issues was extracurricular. They would not have been addressed at any of the SNFs that had been recommended. Not a single clinician told us to do this. And yet fixing his eyes and his teeth seemed primal, integral to returning to life—for his health, for practical reasons, most of all because they were part of him. As with every other piece of his recovery, there was no guarantee of success. But not trying seemed a strange policy, a punishment, an abandonment. If the idea was to bring back his *person*, how could his eyes and teeth be excluded?

Not to mention his hands.

His wrists had been rescued, but when he tried to open his left hand, it looked like a crab, knuckles caving, fingers unable to straighten. His right hand fared slightly better.

The guitar was Jason's instrument. It was how he best expressed himself. He had dedicated his life to playing it. Would he come back from this injury, all but his hands? Would he live, denied the thing he loved above all else?

In the hospitals we had scrambled to save his hands, wrapping them around tennis balls or Sandy Bell's stuffed German shepherd, massaging them, stretching them, kneading them with lotion to keep his skin from flaking off. The contractures had kept pace with our efforts. One step forward, one step back: at best we had kept his hands from becoming much worse.

Now, every morning, Jason flattened putty into a pancake on the kitchen counter, then nudged it forward one finger at a time. He rolled it into a log into which he dug his nails. He wrapped the putty around his fingers like a rope, then opened his fingers against it. ("Break free of the putty!" I would cheer.) He flipped canned tomatoes upside down and back again, then moved them from one end of the counter to the other. He worked anti-arthritis devices—with pulleys and springs and rubber bands—that I found at my beloved Belmont Medical Supply.

"Thumbs up," we'd say, and he'd put a thumb up.

"Table for one." Pointer finger up.

"Peace out, man." Two fingers.

"W for president." Three fingers.

"Four for the cab." Four fingers.

"Halt!" Five fingers, flat palm.

"Bye-bye." A wave.

"Live long and prosper." Vulcan signature.

And finally, "Fuck you." Up went his middle finger. Fuck you to these exercises. Fuck you to this injury. Fuck you to this long-ass recovery.

These hand exercises belonged to an hour-long post-breakfast workout: first, lying in a giant splint that was opening up his chest while one of us read aloud from the *Times* the tragedy of post-Katrina New Orleans; then stretching and balance and strength exercises prescribed by his therapists, to which we added our own, for example, tongue twisters and making faces in the mirror.

As a musician he understood that practice led to better playing. Running scales and drills had long been part of his daily work. A hard piece could be broken down into sections, each played slowly, then faster, then with the other sections slowly, then faster. The morning regime adhered to the same principle of investing time for a future payoff.

His fingers didn't look like they were changing, but we continued to ask them to push and dig, and we expected that they would, even when they didn't. Equally important to physical change was not sending his fingers the message that they were stuck. As long as there was even the tiniest amount of progress, their recovery continued.

Still, we made an appointment with a renowned hand surgeon.

Rop and I accompanied Jason down a hall lined with framed posters trumpeting teamwork and success to a room where an assistant took X-rays of Jason's hands. After brief introductions the famous doctor explained the surgery, which involved cutting and reattaching a tendon in the forearm. He recommended surgery on both hands.

In the X-rays mounted on the light box, the fingers of Jason's left hand bent so far they looked as if the top two bones had been chopped off.

"What do you think the outcome will be?" we asked.

"I can get the right hand close to normal," the doctor said. "That left hand will never be good for anything."

He told us to stop at the receptionist's desk on our way out to book a surgery date. Then he was gone, barely fifteen minutes after he'd walked in.

"What do you want for your hands?" asked the second surgeon we consulted.

"I want them to be the way they were," Jason said.

For an hour and a half this doctor tested the range of motion for Jason's shoulders, arms, and hands, then asked about Jason's life, his music, the injury, the recovery.

How far did this doctor think Jason's fingers could recover without surgery?

A contemplative, discouraging "Hmm" was all he said at first. But after stretching Jason's fingers, his optimism grew. He offered the same procedure suggested by the first surgeon. He would operate, however, on the left hand only, and even then, he said, "It's a good bit of surgery for one hand." Intense rehabilitation would follow, and Jason might be not better off than he was now. Why not continue with the casts and splints and exercises and come back in three months?

Jason had left the first surgeon's office asking, "What if he's right? What if my left hand is wrecked? What if I can't play?" For the first time in his recovery he'd been told directly *You can't. You won't.*

We weren't looking for doctors to tell us what we wanted to hear. We just wanted doctors who would try. After all, sitting in their examination rooms was a man who not long ago had communicated by blinking. How effortlessly "He'll *probably* never play the guitar again" could become "He'll probably *never* play the guitar again." How easily he might have given up, accepting as prophecy the first doctor's words, "That left hand will never be good for anything."

After seeing the second surgeon, Jason's despair switched to fury. Determined to prove the naysayer wrong, he redoubled his commitment to the tedious exercises and uncomfortable splints.

A second opinion could be the difference not only in treatment but also philosophy—not just the doctor's but Jason's—and for this the first surgeon's words were a gift. They made Jason ask, What do *I* think is possible?

167

His increasing abilities prompted us to recalibrate our routine continuously. Mostly this meant letting him do something he'd previously needed help with, like putting on pants or untying his shoes. Often the recalibration meant getting Muma and Rop to back off. Seeing their son impaired, instinctively they wanted to relieve his suffering. Watching him struggle was painful. In getting his breakfast or clearing his plate, they were being kind, considerate people.

But he was my sibling, my peer, and I bristled at their interventions. They treated him like a child. In some ways he was like a child. He was dependent, needed naps, went to bed around eight, responded well to a structured environment—and he himself was retreading his youth. But he *wasn't* a child.

It didn't matter that it took him longer to get his own glass of water. He could do it, and when he did it again, he became faster and reclaimed that action.

November 14. There is a dangerous temptation to forget that the patient is an adult who has lived independently and made big life choices. More and more, I hear him say, Just give me more time.

Even as we struggled to hit the ever-shifting mark of helping but not too much, sometimes we seemed connected to a strange, magical law of the universe, a higher frequency on which we could bend reality. One Friday afternoon, the date a deadline for prescription coverage—if we missed it, Jason and Monica would be paying out-of-pocket for a month—Jason and I raced to the Mass Health office in Charlestown with paperwork. It was after four. Rush hour was starting. The Mass Health rep took the paperwork, but she needed his ID—driver's license (his had expired) or passport.

"Be right back," we said.

Time stopped as we glided through the thickening traffic, every light green for us, to the apartment, then again through rush hour, riding some kind of wave that dropped us at Mass Health's doorstep at four fifty-seven, where breathlessly we handed over the passport.

Or the morning we flew to Kansas City to see Rop's hundred-year-old mother, Boo. The night before, Monica realized Jason wouldn't get through airport security because she'd mailed his license and passport to Social Security for a replacement for his card, which couldn't be found. At dawn, suitcases loaded in the car, we drove to the Social Security office in Somerville. Already the line stretched down the block. When the doors opened, we took a number, but it was clear that if we waited, we'd miss the flight. I picked a nice-looking woman behind the counter, caught her attention as she paused for something else, explained our situation as briefly as possible.

"Let me check," she said and returned a moment later with Jason's material. "It was just about to be mailed out."

A can-do electricity ran between Monica, Muma, Rop, Jason, and me. Just to watch him while remembering where he'd been a year ago was to know that in a given moment more possibilities existed than were usually acknowledged. The wellspring of our super-expansion being months of terrible fear, we drank deep of these moments, feeling briefly the giddy invincibility of the sole survivors of a shipwreck.

30

In the beginning was the question of life or death, and the hospitals had kept Jason alive. Then came the question of movement and speech, and Spaulding had revived his ability to move and speak. Now his recovery addressed the everything-else of his injury, whose tentacles had reached the furthest points of his existence. Now he faced the question of restoring who he was.

One night in early December, amid the half-unpacked boxes, Jason picked up a Stratocaster. From across the basement I watched him. Bent over the guitar, he looked like he was testing it as one would when considering an instrument for purchase.

Since his days in the hospital, I had known that I would never help him with this. I would never broach the subject of playing. If the desire and ability were there, so be it. If not, I would love him no less.

Still, seeing him pick up the guitar, I was ecstatic.

He wasn't. The contractures in his hands made playing unbearably painful. He didn't last five minutes.

He'd had blue spells before this, but now a heaviness descended, as if his weight had suddenly doubled. Everything became harder, slower, longer. His shoulders drooped. His already precarious posture sagged. Like a flu, the gloom consumed him.

Dr. Carter said the depression was, paradoxically, a good sign. It meant Jason was processing what had happened to him. The alternative—that he remain unaware of his injury and impairments—was worse. But I worried that after this great effort to keep him alive, to return him to life, he might end it. At least suicide would be his choice. He had thought about how he would do it, I heard him tell a doctor—his memory still faulty, I sat in on his appointments—but he wouldn't because he couldn't leave Ellie with that legacy.

Besides his inability to play, he was realizing that he had missed Ellie's birth. Since he'd come home he had been spending time with her almost every day but without feeling an emotional connection. It was dawning on him: *She's my daughter. I missed the pregnancy. I missed her birth. She's already nine months old.*

From our perspective he was a man who had not only beaten death but had gone from mute immobility to writing essays for his speech therapist about how to produce an album. But for him every aspect of his life was disturbingly unfamiliar: he was stiff, weak, dizzy, foggy, tired, a grown man whose parents, wife, and sister helped him with the most basic tasks. We'd had months to accept the bleed and complications, to transition from shock to action. He was just now starting to understand what had happened—plus, he was the guy it had happened to. There was no break from it. We couldn't have been closer, but the injury was his alone.

I stuck to the routine, wishing to come across as solid, steady, reliable.

If progress was the plateau, he would continue making progress. He would change and get better.

Whether that applied to his spirit remained to be seen.

Between therapy appointments we were Christmas shopping. Loud and visually crazy, the atmosphere of the stores scrambled his signals. We retreated outside, regrouped, reentered. As he approached the cash register for the first time, I hung back, watching for signs of miscommunication or confusion. The deftness with which he pulled his credit card from his wallet and signed the slip surprised me. Of all the actions he'd relearned, this one resurfaced with an almost automaton precision, the exchange playing like an experiment sponsored by a bank to survey the neurological map of its consumers.

That night he asked me, "If the weather isn't too bad tomorrow, would you be up for more Christmas shopping?"

"Do you know where you want to go?"

"Newbury Street."

We went to Newbury Street.

It helped that he knew Boston. His freshman year had been at the Berklee College of Music, and he'd played hundreds of gigs in the local clubs. Not only did he know neighborhoods and geography, he knew local musicians.

"Are you playing out at all?" asked Duke Levine when he visited.

"Not really," Jason replied. "Everything I do is for my recovery."

Every week his friends came, and though his end of the conversation was sparse, he would say over and over how nice it was that they had made the trip, how good it was to see them. Later he would say he was "less aware of the person than of a kind of aura."

December 17. Monica started a great discussion about helping Jason with Ellie. I got bagels and chai at 1369, and we stood around in the kitchen talking and laughing while Jay toasted the bagels. He says he feels more with-it today, less out of it. First time he's said this.

"It's coming faster," Peter told him. "You had your own thought process, and you were able to block me out when I wasn't being helpful."

With the PT near but not touching him, Jason walked up and down the hallway on his own.

A week before my birthday, he asked Muma if she had anything planned.

He was working doggedly, day in, day out, never without the problems with his hands and eyes, never escaping the fatigue that came over him like waves. Living with all of us, every moment geared to his recovery, I thought he must have cabin fever. Or maybe I was thinking of myself.

After Christmas, Muma, Jason, and I drove to a little town in New Hampshire's White Mountains. It was only a few hours from Cambridge, but the immense evergreens and head-high mounds of snow let us believe we'd gone a great distance.

Sleigh ride on a frigid night, hot tub in a tower overlooking Mount Washington, lattés in a flower store–cum–coffee shop: these would be the first memories that he could hold onto since getting into an ambulance sixteen months earlier.

"What was the name of the town?" a friend asked a few days after we'd returned. My mind went blank, wiped clean by exhaustion and stress.

But Jason remembered: "Franconia."

Weekday mornings Rop would pick up the *Times* at a nearby market. In January Jason said he wanted to get the paper. Alone.

I pictured the two and a half blocks between the apartment and the store. He would have to cross a street. Could he see well enough to make sure a driver or cyclist wasn't barreling through a red light? Would he be aware of someone coming up behind him? How would he protect himself?

All right, we said.

As soon as Jason was out the door, Rop turned to me. "Should I follow him?"

"I don't know," I said. I understood his impulse, but in agreeing to let Jason go, I had decided to trust whatever benevolent spirits had protected him thus far. We had helped him back to life, and part of life was risk.

Rop put on his coat and left. Five minutes later he hurried in, hung his coat in the closet, and sat down on the couch next to me.

"I don't think he saw me," he said.

A minute later Jason walked in with the paper, beaming.

Combing through old computer files—which he was reviewing just as he was retracing every other item from his previous life—Jason came across an unfinished project, an album he'd been producing from songs that had been recorded but not used on the sophomore album of Goats in Trees, Jason's band with Monica, Jeff Hill, and John Mettam. After transferring the two-inch tape to Pro Tools, Jason had stripped the vocal tracks. Then, on a whim, he'd invited Amy Correia to sing one of the songs. Thrilled with the result, he had asked Teddy Thompson to sing a song. Another success. With the sardonic notion of making a tribute album to himself, he began asking various performers to sing his songs. He'd recorded a handful—then was interrupted by the bleed.

Playing the guitar was torture, but completing the album gave him purpose beyond the long winter slog of doctors and therapies and exercises. He had to consider whose voice would fit the unfinished songs; contact people and ask them to sing; schedule their sessions in his studio, in which the number of moving boxes was gradually dwindling; update his software and prepare the studio for recording the new tracks; then oversee mixing, mastering, artwork, pressing.

He undertook the assignment as a mission upon which depended his real recovery. Walk, talk, eat, shower, dress—yes. But music was, as it had always been, his truth.

With her parents sharing Ellie's child care, Monica returned to work. Addis and Diane, no longer needed to help Jason with his morning routine, stopped coming. Instead of going to swim therapy, Jason, Muma, and I frequented the pool at MIT. He wore a floatation belt and needed direction on what to do next, but he was swimming in the pool like everyone else.

No longer dependent, he was not yet independent. Like body-guards, we shadowed him. With his eyesight still compromised, we were his transportation. Nights I went with him to open mikes, where he introduced himself to local musicians and made contacts as he'd done years ago when he was starting out.

"Such a drag that I have to do all this again," he would say. Nevertheless, he was doing it.

The role my parents and I had played was evaporating. After a year and a half of intense hands-on involvement, now mostly we watched, but stepping back left us dislocated. Muma would cook all weekend, which gave us delicious food for most of the week, but her activity was infused with a crazed energy, the need to go all-out, a sense that anything less than exhaustion wasn't adequate.

"Do you want me to cut up some strawberries for you?" Rop asked Jason one morning as Jason poured himself a bowl of cereal.

"Jason can do it," I said.

"I'm just thinking of *time*, Marjorie," Rop replied.

When you have different names and someone who usually calls you by a nickname uses your full name, you know it's code for something else—usually anger, which I recognized because I too was angry: burned-out from going nonstop every day, from fighting for Jason, from stress, from having my own work and life paused for so long. The amount of time my parents and I could live together had passed its expiration date. We were curdling.

In late March, Teddy Thompson called. He was coming to Boston to play a show at the Paradise and wanted to know if Jason would sit in on a song.

No sooner had Jason hung up the phone than he started practicing, but other factors were more troublesome. His balance wasn't dependable. His sense of space was skewed. The double vision sometimes tricked him into missing steps or edges. Done with catheters, still when he went out, he wore the bulky and uncomfortable weird underwear. Sudden, intense fatigue often left him no choice but to lie down. The show would start at ten; he'd been going to sleep around eight.

Monica, Rop, and I went with Jason to the club. We walked into the large empty room, then Jason turned and headed through a door leading backstage.

"Jason!" the guys in the band shouted when they saw him.

I could see on Monica and Rop's faces exactly what I felt—feigned offense at how easily he'd deserted us, joy to see him in his element.

The club filled and the show began. After a few songs Teddy introduced Jason, and he came out, stumbled for a step, righted himself, picked up the guitar.

He was back onstage, returned to the place where he'd fallen.

The next day Monica and Ellie moved in with Jason, and I moved into my own apartment, taking over a lease for a woman returning home to help her father. I had a few months to decide whether to renew the lease—whether to stay.

The gig with Teddy cracked open Jason's depression. He began practicing daily, determined to rebuild his stamina and fix his hands. With an occupational therapist who specialized in helping musicians, he made a careful plan for increasing his playing time. As for his hands, he could work on them, through exercises and splints, and he could work around them. He switched the neck on his favorite guitar for one with a grip that suited him better. Unable to see his pedals—for various effects, for example, the wah-wah—he moved them from the floor to a table and hit their switches with his hand instead of his foot. He found alternate chord fingerings. When he couldn't get his slide over his left pinkie's knuckle, Rop had the hardware store cut an archway in a short metal tube, then fitted it with Velcro.

He played a few songs with Richard Julian at Club Passim. A set with Amy Correia. A Lizard Lounge show with Dennis Brennan. Preparing for and getting through each performance required a monumental effort, but he delivered, rewarded each time with a rush of triumph.

But he wasn't connecting to the music. "No clams," as he put it, but he didn't feel he was contributing. Primarily an improviser, now he was just playing the songs.

Rachel Loshak asked him to join her at the Living Room in New York. Jason had performed in this club thousands of times. In its sound booth had hung, for nearly two years, a picture of him, under which someone had scratched, "GIT BACK CRIGLER." The giddy, happy homecoming was standing room only, and after the encore the crowd sang to him. It was his birthday.

At last something clicked. Not only did he feel connected to the music, but the experience of playing became more immediate, as if the distance between his mind and hands had shortened. The old critical voice was gone, replaced by a new freedom—"a riskier use of space," he would accurately describe his playing—an exploration directly informed by the restrictions he'd endured and overcome.

I had always thought of the Living Room as opposed to, say, the dining room. That night I got it: the place where we are alive.

His medical recovery would last several more years.

There would be another round of proton beam radiation treatment on the AVM, which would shrink to oblivion.

Two surgeries on his eyes to correct the strabismus, plus massive amounts of vision therapy.

Palate expansion surgery, teeth extraction, braces.

Dozens more splints on his fingers—but never surgery.

Therapeutic exercise gave way to exercise.

He retook driver's ed—because he'd had a handicap placard—renewed his license, and started driving again.

He pursued acupuncture and biofeedback to treat the overwhelming fatigue that debilitated him more than anything. He sought ways to feel productive and healthy and good. "It's all a state of mind," he would tell himself when he got down. He practiced focusing on what he had, what he could be grateful for, letting go of what he'd missed, what he lacked.

He took on the project of his recovery, which is to say he took on his life, the power to determine the course of his day, which was what, all along, we had wished for him.

His outpatient work at Spaulding would wind down to occasional sessions for the therapists to measure how far his contracted joints had opened up. Years after his injury the joints were still opening.

The price for his recovery would total about $3.5 million, a fraction of what it would have cost for him to spend the rest of his life in some kind of facility. Three and a half million dollars later, he returned to his life and work. He was performing, scoring films and commercials, and he finished and released the tribute album *The Music of Jason Crigler*.

Gradually, we settled back into being a normal family, whatever that is—at any rate, not a family in crisis. Phone calls were not about Jason's emergencies or triumphs but to share news, like Ellie starting nursery school, to which Jason brought her every morning.

In January 2007, at last, Jason would remember a year ago, a time he would describe as the beginning of his life.

31

Before I could unpack in my new apartment, Muma's father, Lyman, died.

Lyman had been born in Walla Walla, Washington, to parents whose parents had moved there from the Oregon Territory. Except for his time in the navy—as a Seabee during World War II he laid landing strips in the Pacific; later he served in Korea—Lyman worked exclusively for California's Department of Highways. Even when he'd forgotten who I was, he could tell me about the first public talks on construction of the Santa Monica Freeway. His mother, Marjorie, had helped raise my mother. I came to know Lyman and my grandmother Burris first when I was at Stanford and then after, while living in San Francisco and Los Angeles. He was my connection to the West, to ancestors who had fought in the Revolutionary War, to the meaning behind my name.

I flew to Carmel for the memorial service. Standing in a hotel room looking out at the wet lush green, the cypress trees, the Santa Lucia Mountains, I knew what I would do.

California had been a refuge for me in the past. It could be that once more.

Come back, said the salt air and night-blooming jasmine.

I needed to be in a place that spoke to me spiritually, where I felt peaceful. In August I moved. Crossing the Bay Bridge my first night in, I knew I'd been fooling myself, that the move had been a mistake.

I stayed almost a year, then returned East, moving three more times before landing in western Massachusetts, which held me while finally I started to decompress.

I did need a place that was peaceful, spiritual, but it wasn't to be found on a map.

When the questions had concerned life or death, my days had had a strangely seductive simplicity. Returning to the banality of ordinary existence was crushing. Accustomed to crisis, I revved too high, still hypervigilant, grinding my teeth at night, as out of practice socially as someone who'd spent two years as a desert hermit. Every decision was affected by the urgent knowledge that I could die at any moment, and while awareness of death helps make a meaningful life, so does emptying the moving boxes. Temporary homes became too much a habit, as did undertaking projects that depleted me but kept me from coming down from the frenzied energy of the crisis.

I didn't want to know what I would find when I sat still. So many emotions had been denied every time I walked into Jason's hospital room. I tried to discard them without examination.

The sorrow had to come out.

Many times I had looked at Jason and other patients and thought, This kind of injury is a sad part of life.

It is one thing to think, *This is sad.* It is another to feel it.

When I finally stopped moving, I cried and cried. The pain spilled out of me. Even though my parents and Monica and I had always believed Jason was there, for a while we'd lost him. We had lived too long not knowing if he would come back or how far: too long parched, drinking water in droplets.

A part of me had been set aside. Reclaiming it was messy, clumsy, chaotic. Stunted, I had to learn again how to be a reciprocal friend, how to work for someone else. I had to learn again faith, a faith not centered on Jason.

At the same time, I had a bedrock sense of relief and satisfaction, for I had heard the call and answered it.

This was the story: a hemorrhage in my brother's brain failed to kill him.

When we are in danger, sometimes we get lucky and circumstances leave a narrow path out. Sometimes other people save us. And sometimes we survive by saying, This can be done.

In our summers at the yellow house on Lake Hayward, Jason and I would swim—leaning on heavy black inner tubes—to the small public beach on the far shore. We went to the beach for its sand. Near our house the lake bottom was mud as soft as yogurt, with long tickling grass and twigs that poked my feet.

We were at that beach when an afternoon thunderstorm rolled in. The crowd scattered, people gathering blankets and chairs as quickly as if they were in a race.

"Let's walk," I said, picturing us on the shoulder of the asphalt road, barefoot, in our bathing suits, carrying inner tubes.

"Let's swim," Jason said.

In the torrential rain my body above the water felt the same as my body below, and the din of the downpour drowned out the thunder, but I could see lightning's pale lines flash in the white sky. Jason took us into the storm. What choice did I have but to follow? Kicking hard, we swam into the tempest, as if only by going straight into it, only by going all the way in, could we reach home.

To order or obtain more information on these or other University of Nebraska Press titles, visit nebraskapress.unl.edu.